# THE PLAN

# EAT WELL, LOSE WEIGHT, TRANSFORM YOUR LIFE

## AOIFE HEARNE (RD)

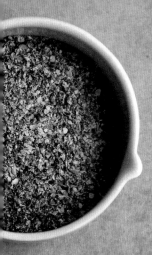

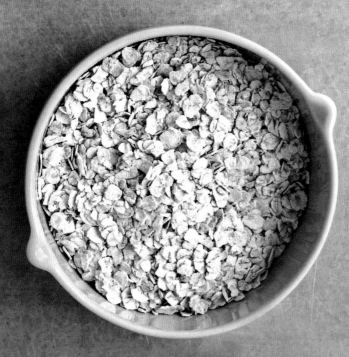

Gill Books

To Alan, Dylan and Alva ... my taste testers!

**Gill Books**
Hume Avenue
Park West
Dublin 12
www.gillbooks.ie

Gill Books is an imprint of M.H. Gill and Co.

© Aoife Hearne 2016

978 07171 7092 0

Designed by www.grahamthew.com
Photography © Joanne Murphy www.joanne-murphy.com
Styled by Orla Neligan of Cornershop Productions www.cornershopproductions.com
Assisted by Jane Flanagan

PROPS
Avoca: HQ Kilmacanogue, Bray, Co Wicklow.
T: (01) 2746939; E: info@avoca.ie;
W: www.avoca.ie
•••
Meadows & Byrne: Dublin, Cork, Galway, Clare, Tipperary.
T: (01) 2804554/(021) 4344100; E: info@meadowsandbyrne.ie;
W: www.meadowsandbyrne.com
•••
Marks & Spencer: Unit 1 - 28, Dundrum Town Centre, Dublin 16.
T: (01) 299 1300; W: www.marksandspencer.ie
•••
Article Dublin: Powerscourt Townhouse, South William Street, Dublin 2.
T: (01) 6799268; E: items@articledublin.com; W: www.articledublin.com
•••
Dunnes Stores: 46-50 South Great Georges Street, Dublin 2.
T: 1890 253185; W: www.dunnesstores.com
•••
Harold's Bazaar: 208 Harold's Cross Road, Dublin 6W.
T: 087 7228789.
•••
Historic Interiors: Oberstown, Lusk, Co Dublin.
T: (01) 8437174; E: killian@historicinteriors.net
•••
TK Maxx: The Park, Carrickmines, Dublin 18.
T: (01) 2074798; W: www.tkmaxx.ie
•••
Golden Biscotti ceramics.
W: http://goldenbiscotti.bigcartel.com
•••
The Patio Centre: The Hill Centre, Johnstown Road, Glenageary, Cabinteely, Dublin 18.
T: 01 2350714; W: thepatiocentre.com
•••
Industry Design: 41 A/B Drury Street, Dublin 2.
T: (01) 6139111; W: industrydesign.ie

Indexed by Eileen O'Neill
Printed by Printer Trento Srl, Italy

This book is typeset in 10 on 14pt Clavo.

*The paper used in this book comes from the wood pulp of managed forests. For every tree
felled, at least one tree is planted, thereby renewing natural resources.*

A CIP catalogue record for this book is available from the British Library.

5 4 3 2

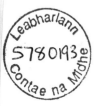

# The Plan

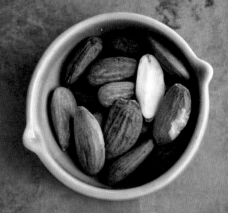

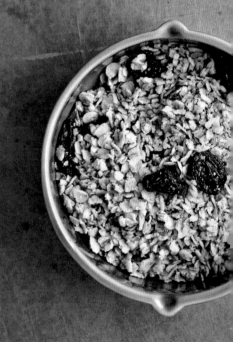

## About the Author

Aoife Hearne is a registered dietitian, a member of the Irish Nutrition and Dietetic Institute, the professional body for dietitians in Ireland, and a member of the dietitians' registration board of CORU, Ireland's multi-profession health regulator. Aoife studied nutrition at the University of Tennessee on an athletics scholarship and went on to complete a dietetic internship at the world-renowned Massachusetts General Hospital, Boston. Aoife has been the nutrition expert on RTÉ's *Operation Transformation* since 2014 and was the first dietitian to be part of the show in the year it won an IFTA. She lives in Waterford with her husband and family.

# ACKNOWLEDGEMENTS

I would like to thank Sarah Liddy of Gill Books for the interest she showed in this book from the very start and for the great support through the process of making my ideas for this book become a reality. I would like to thank Ruth Mahony and Aoife O'Kelly for their great editorial support.

A big thanks to Orla Neligan and Jo Murphy for your attention to detail with the photography and making the pictures of my meals look so much better than when I serve them at home!

A sincere thanks to my friend and colleague Niamh O'Connor, dietitian, who has been a great mentor since starting my private practice in 2005. Thanks also to Michelle Lane, dietitian, who worked tirelessly on the nutrition analysis for these recipes and endured the many changes from beginning to end.

To my wonderful colleagues and friends in the *Operation Transformation* family – thanks for all the support and laughs over the past few years. Karl, Ciara and Eddie, you have made something that is technically classified as 'work' a very fun experience. Thanks to the leaders for their bravery in sharing their stories with us and the nation. To Philip, Niamh, Steven, Sinead and Grainne of Vision Independent Productions and RTÉ, joint makers of Operation Transformation, thanks for giving me the opportunity to present a non-diet approach to healthy eating to the nation.

To my friends, both in Ireland and the US, thanks for your support, wisdom and taste-testing skills!

I would like to thank the extended Kirwan family for the encouragement they have given me since joining the Kirwan clan. In particular, thanks to my mother-in-law (Granny Brid) for sharing some of her recipes and cooking experiences with me.

I would like to thank my parents, Martin and Corinne, who have been my constant support system from the very start! It's hard to put into words how much I appreciate the support and love you have shown me and how that has shaped me into the person I am today.

Last, but by no means least – thanks to my husband Alan for his love, patience and belief in me and our two adorable babies, Dylan and Alva. I am so grateful for the life we have together.

# Contents

A little bit about me ................................................ 2
How to use this book ............................................ 6
A little bit about the recipes ............................. 24
Weekly plans ......................................................... 25

## BREAKFAST
## QUICK AND EASY BREAKFASTS
Porridge and Fruit ................................................ 30
Boiled Egg and English Muffin ......................... 32
Overnight Oats ..................................................... 33
Breakfast Sandwich .............................................. 35
Berry and Chia Smoothie .................................. 36

## WEEKEND BREAKFAST TREATS
Hot Start ................................................................ 37
Continental Fruit Salad ...................................... 38
Omelette ................................................................ 39
    Mushroom and Ricotta ................................. 39
    Mixed Pepper ................................................. 39
    Goat's Cheese and Spinach ........................ 39
    Bacon and Tomato ........................................ 39
Mini Grill ............................................................... 40
Tropical Muesli Cup ........................................... 42
Mediterranean Breakfast Pitta ........................ 45
Cinnamon and Yogurt Pancakes ................... 46
French Toast ......................................................... 49

## LUNCH
## SUPER SANDWICHES
Base and Filling ................................................... 52
Hot Chicken .......................................................... 54
Chicken Salad ...................................................... 54

Baked Ham and Cheese ............................................................ 55
Turkey Club .............................................................................. 55
Salmon and Dill Mayo .............................................................. 56
Mid-Week Lunch-Time Staples: Soup and Sandwiches ........ 58

## SOULFUL SOUPS
Chicken Noodle Soup ............................................................... 60
Sweet Potato and Celery Soup ................................................ 61
Butternut Squash and Vegetable Soup .................................... 62
Cream of Broccoli Soup ............................................................ 63
Minestrone Soup ...................................................................... 65
Carrot and Coriander Soup ...................................................... 66
Hearty Chickpea Soup .............................................................. 68
Chicken and Lentil Soup .......................................................... 70
Pea and Mint Soup ................................................................... 71

## SASSY SALADS
Tempting Turkey Salad and Crisp Bread ................................. 74
Tantalising Tuna Salad ............................................................. 75
BBQ Chicken Salad ................................................................... 78
Tuna Panzanella Salad ............................................................. 79
Sunshine Salad ......................................................................... 80
Caprese Pasta Salad ................................................................. 83
Tomato and Avocado Salad ...................................................... 84
Spinach Salad with Chicken, Corn and Feta ............................ 85
Baked Tomatoes with Goat's Cheese ....................................... 86
Cajun-Grilled Chicken and Black-Eyed Bean Salad ............... 88

## DINNER
### BEEF
Lasagne and Salad .................................................................... 92
Curry Beef Noodle Bowl .......................................................... 94
Spaghetti Bolognese ................................................................ 96
Ginger Beef .............................................................................. 97
Cottage Pie .............................................................................. 99
Beef and Rice ........................................................................... 100

Italian Steak ......................................................... 102
Meatballs and Spaghetti .................................. 103
Pot Roast ............................................................ 104
Chilli .................................................................... 105
Beef Lo Mein ..................................................... 108
Buffalo Steak and Corn ................................... 109

## FISH

Sea Bass with Salsa-Inspired Sauce ............... 110
Mexican Cod ...................................................... 112
Sun-Dried Tomato Salmon ............................... 114
Salmon and Couscous ....................................... 115
Quick Fish Stew ................................................. 117
Quick Tuna Pasta .............................................. 118
Seafood Curry .................................................... 119
Mackerel and Quinoa ....................................... 120
Haddock with Coconut Rice ............................ 122
Teriyaki Salmon and Coriander Rice ............. 123
Chilli Salmon Noodle Bowl ............................. 126
Indian Fish Curry .............................................. 127
Fish Cakes and Salad ........................................ 128
Curry Coconut Fish Parcel ............................... 131

## PORK

Pork Tenderloin with Orange Marinade ......... 132
Spicy Pork and Carrot Stir-Fry ....................... 134
Sweet and Sour Pork ........................................ 135
Pork Medallions with Super Green Sauce ..... 137
Pork with Sprouts ............................................. 138
Pork Steak with Peppers and Creamy Polenta ........ 139

## POULTRY

Chicken and Chorizo Pasta Bake .................... 140
Herby Roast Chicken ........................................ 143
Chicken and Loaded-Vegetable Bake ............. 144
Mango Chicken ................................................... 145
Chicken and Ginger Curry ............................... 146
Chicken Fajitas .................................................. 148

Chicken Quesadillas and Salad ....................................................... 149
Spanish Chicken ...................................................................................152
Stuffed Chicken with Lemon, Capers and Chilli .................... 153
Granny Brid's Chicken ...................................................................... 154
Tex Mex Chicken and Wholewheat Noodles ........................... 156
Roast Basil Chicken ........................................................................... 157
Five-Spice Chicken ............................................................................ 158
Roast Italian-Style Spicy Chicken ............................................... 159
Spanish Chicken Stew with Chickpeas ...................................... 161
Chicken Parmesan ............................................................................. 162
Grilled Chicken and Sweetcorn Salad with Chilli
    Cream Dressing ........................................................................... 163
Turkey Pesto Pasta ........................................................................... 164

## LITTLE HELPERS

Fish Goujons ......................................................................................... 166
Chicken Goujons ................................................................................. 167
Chicken Kebabs ................................................................................... 170
Veggie Pancakes ................................................................................. 172

## MEATLESS MONDAY

Protein Substitutes ........................................................................... 173
Goat's Cheese and Beetroot Salad ............................................. 174
Smoked Mozzarella Couscous Salad .......................................... 176
Pepper Frittata ................................................................................... 177
Falafel ..................................................................................................... 180
Butternut Squash and Lentil Curry ............................................ 182
Punchy Pasta and Roasted Tomatoes ....................................... 183
Creamy Mushroom Pasta ............................................................... 185
Courgette and Corn Chilli .............................................................. 186
Moroccan Chickpea Stew ............................................................... 187

## SATURDAY TAKEAWAY MEALS

Sizzling Steak Fajitas ....................................................................... 188
Hawaiian-Inspired Chicken Fingers and Sweet
    Potato Wedges ............................................................................. 190
Chicken Tacos ..................................................................................... 193
Fish Pie ................................................................................................... 194

Thai Red Curry and Fried Rice ................................... 195
Cheesy Nachos ................................................... 196
Saturday Night Pizza Special ................................... 199
Beef with Mushroom Sauce and Sweet Potato Wedges ...... 200
Cheeseburger and Fries ......................................... 201
Veggie Burger .................................................. 202

## SALAD DRESSINGS AND SAUCES

The Best Tomato-Based Sauce ................................... 206
Sweet and Sour Sauce .......................................... 207
Vinaigrette Salad Dressing .................................... 209
Taco Spice Mix ................................................ 210
Fajita Spice Mix .............................................. 210

## SNACKS

Smoked Salmon Roll ............................................ 214
Crackers and Cheese ........................................... 214
Fruit Cup ..................................................... 215
Fruit and Nuts ................................................ 216
Veggies and Hummus ............................................ 219
Spinach and Mango Smoothie .................................... 220
Beetroot and Orange Smoothie .................................. 222
Baked Berry Squares ........................................... 223

Nutritional Information Per Serving ........................... 226
Index ......................................................... 238

comhairle chontae na mí
*meath county council*

Meath County Libraries
Dunshaughlin

### Customer name: McMahon, Margaret
### Customer ID: **********5307

### Items that you have renewed

Title: All sewn up : 35 exquisite projects using
appliqué, embroidery, and more
ID: 30011007133557
**Due: Wednesday 12 October 2022**

Title: How to quilt and patchwork: with over
100 techniques and 15 easy projects
ID: 30011006679626
**Due: Wednesday 12 October 2022**

Title: Over My Dead Body
ID: 30011008164742
**Due: Wednesday 12 October 2022**

Title: Takedown
ID: 30011006708524
**Due: Wednesday 12 October 2022**


Total items: 4
Borrow 7
Overdue: 0
Hold requests: 0
Ready for collection: 0
21/09/2022 12:07

### Items that you already have on loan

Title: Learn to cook with Neven : get it right first
time
ID: 30011008165152
**Due: Wednesday 12 October 2022**

Title: Neven Maguire's home economics for life
ID: 30011007136550
**Due: Wednesday 12 October 2022**

Title: The plan : eat well, lose weight, transform
your life
ID: 30011005780193
**Due: Wednesday 12 October 2022**


Thank you for using the SelfCheck System.

Customer ID: **********5301


ID: 3001100713357

ID: 3001100670628

ID: 3001100164742

ID: 3001100670524

21/09/2022 2.07


ID: 3001100713665 0

ID: 3001100576019 5

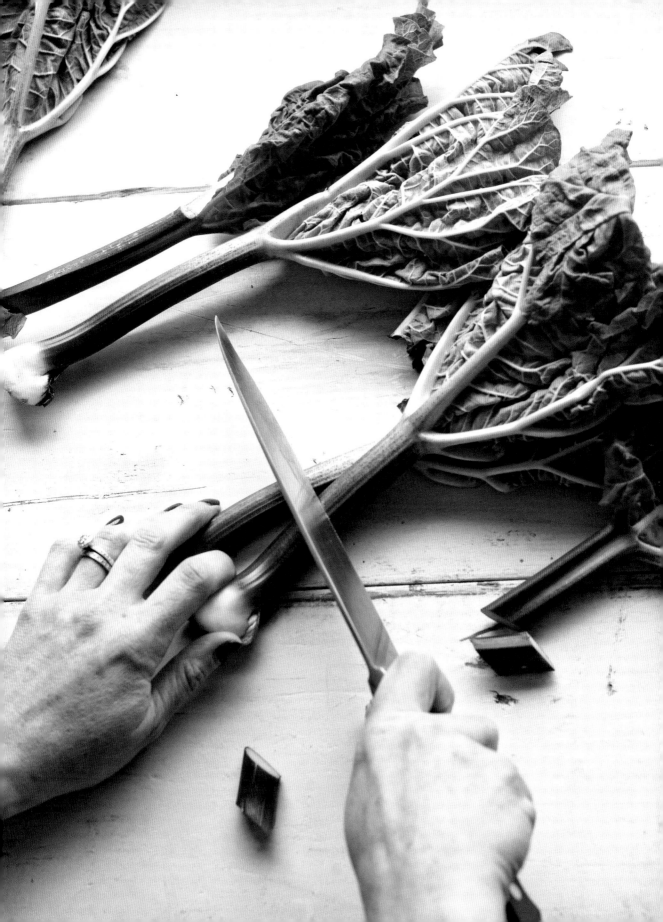

# A LITTLE BIT ABOUT ME

Having trained and worked as a dietitian in the United States for almost eight years, I returned to my home city of Waterford in 2005 and set up my own private practice. My first consultation took place in a converted room in my parents' house, and I could hardly imagine how my career was going to take off! That first client referred seven more and things went from there. From those humble beginnings, my private practice has gone from strength to strength and brought me to the national stage.

In 2014 I joined the *Operation Transformation* team as the nutrition expert on the panel. It was certainly a daunting task at first, but with great support from my co-experts and the production team, it has been such an enjoyable and rewarding experience. It is great to be involved in something that has such a positive impact on the health of our nation. My role on the show is to devise the recipes and guide our leaders and the nation in the right direction for eating well and losing weight. Year in, year out, the show proves that the plan works and, even better, it works for the long term. The plan is very simple: eat better foods, eat appropriate portions, move more!

The most rewarding feeling is meeting previous leaders years later and seeing that they have continued with the plan; that they have maintained the weight they lost and continue to lose more, striving for a healthier weight. The changes to their eating habits and attitude to exercise have had a positive impact not only on their lives, but also on their families and communities. It has been a great learning experience, and much of what I have learned over my years on the show, including the recipes, is here in this book.

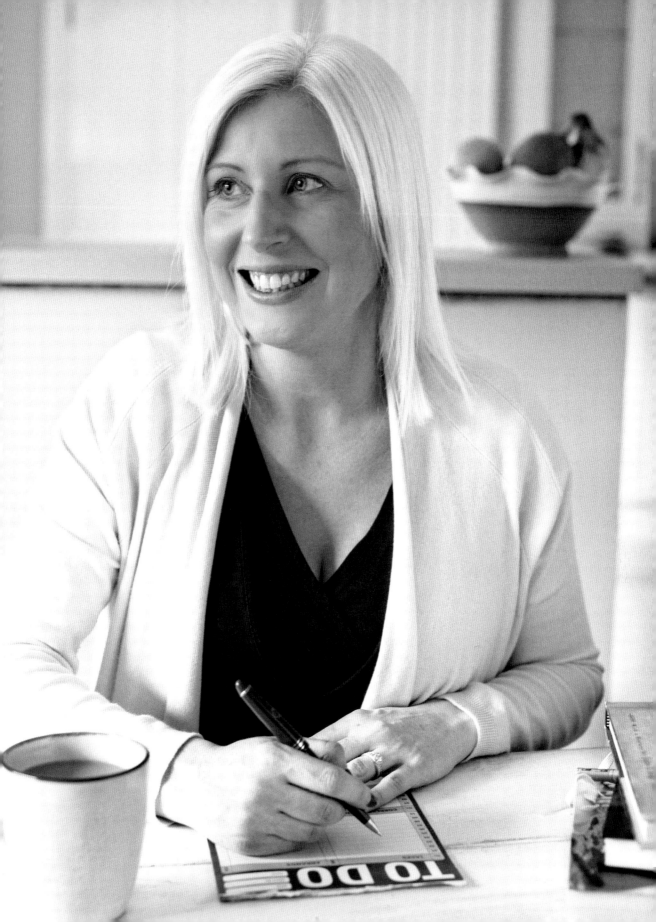

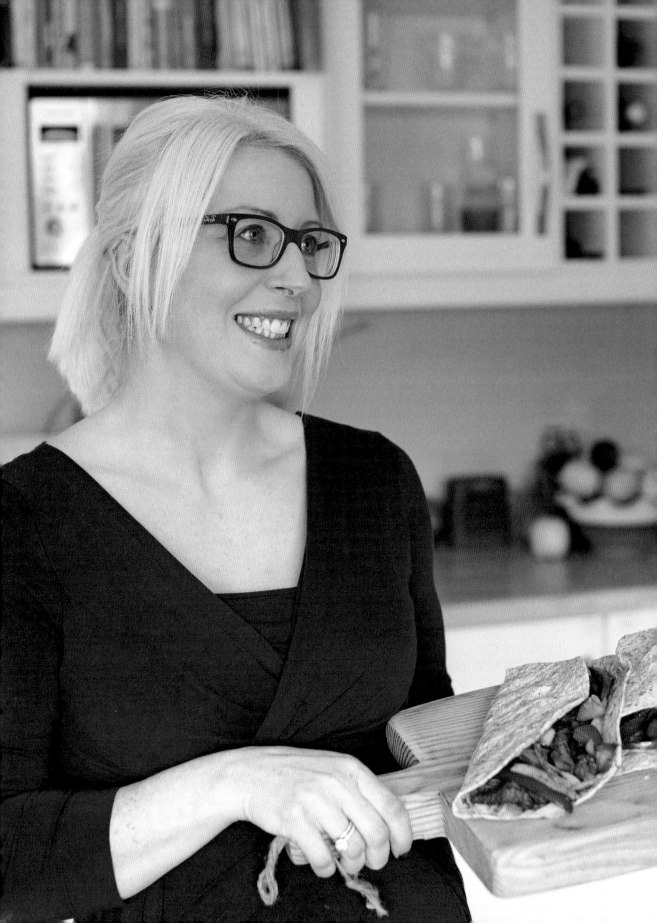

There is a great saying, 'Do what you love and you'll never work a day in your life.' I truly believe this and I have to say I LOVE what I do. It never feels like a chore when I'm working with people who want to make changes to their lifestyle, be it one to one, in a group setting or in the media.

Becoming a mother for the first time in 2014 shaped me in a way I could never have imagined. It was about this time I became passionate about supporting pregnant women and families, and how powerful this can be to change the health of our nation for the better. When my little boy Dylan turned six months, we started to introduce solids, and it made me start thinking about how I was cooking and how I would have to adjust things going forward. I am a strong believer in 'one family, one meal', so I knew if I was going to practise what I preach, there were going to have to be some changes!

I learn so much from the clients I work with – be they in my clinic, the sporting field or the corporate setting. The one thing I know for sure is that in each of these settings, the key to success is about getting the simple things right and being persistent with them. Perfection is really not required, but it is about making the healthy choice the easy choice.

I hope there are recipes here that will become family favourites, just like they are in my family. Life is for living and food is to be enjoyed, and that is something we shouldn't forget!

xoxo

# HOW TO USE THIS BOOK

Let me be clear – in case you are under any illusions – this is NOT a diet book. However, fear not, this book is here to help you and your family make lifelong changes to improve your food choices and to lose weight.

Over the past 10 years or so in my clinic, and especially over the past few years on TV, I have found that the people who are most successful at losing weight long term are those who embraced making a complete change to their lifestyle and who avoided the pitfalls of falling into a yo-yo dieting pattern.

My intention with this book is that you will start to think a little differently about how you eat, what you eat, when you eat and why you eat. I want to help you to be successful at making better meal choices for you and your family and, in turn, to lose weight if that is your goal.

## WHAT IS THE BEST APPROACH FOR WEIGHT LOSS?

Most people don't know how to focus on losing weight without going on a diet. Did you know that only 2% of people lose weight successfully when following a diet? The thing is, diets don't work. In fact, most people who follow diets will actually regain more weight than they lost in the first place. So this book gives you an opportunity to take a different approach. That approach is to focus on wellness and lifestyle changes. Instead of focusing on avoiding certain foods, you are placing your focus on the bigger picture of changing your habits and behaviours to make weight loss stick.[1] Much of current research suggests that this approach

1 Mann, T. *et al.* (2007), 'Medicare's search for effective obesity treatments: Diets are not the answer', *American Psychologist*, vol. 62(3), April 2007, 220–233.

will be more beneficial for you and your family in the long term.

**'Just tell me what I need to do!' My top 5 tips**
Sound familiar? Yes, because this is what most people want – I regularly hear 'just tell me what I need to do and I'll do it'. The first important step is to make sure your head is in the right place so that you can get off to the best start. These are some starter tips, but you will notice other tips along the way to build up your toolbox.

1 Have a strong foundation for WHY you want to lose weight/make changes. This needs to be something that resonates with your soul, a reason strong enough to stop you having two biscuits on the way up the stairs to bed.
2 Be honest with yourself. If you really want to be successful in maintaining a healthy weight for life, you need to stop believing the 'line' you are telling everyone around you. For example, 'I overeat because I'm lonely/I'm sad/I'm bored'; the list can go on. Or instead of the line 'I'm too busy to cook', the truth may be closer to I'm not organised/ prepared at the weekends to be able to cook mid-week and I don't want to take the time needed to do this.
3 Make the healthy habits EASY to do. Think of the 'triggers' that make the healthy habits/food choices easy to do. For example, if you want to drink more water, rather than focusing on drinking 2 litres of water a day, what I recommend is to keep the focus on bringing a water bottle with you to work. If you have your water bottle with you (the trigger), you are more likely to achieve your goal (healthy habit).
4 Build barriers to unhealthy habits. Make it difficult to continue the unhealthy habits that get in the way of your weight loss goals.
5 Make sure you are not on a 'diet'. Keep your focus on the habits you want to change rather than on an 'all or nothing' approach.

**But seriously, what do I need to do?**

Okay – now over to the practical tips and tricks to get you started:

- Keep a food diary. Although very tedious and boring at times, food diaries do work. Research shows that people who keep a food diary lose almost twice as much weight as those who don't.
- Eat regularly. Make sure you never skip meals, especially breakfast. My recommendation is to eat three main meals (breakfast, lunch and dinner) each day, in addition to two snacks.
- Get your five-a-day. This very basic advice – but there is not a person on the planet who is overweight or obese from eating too much broccoli. Make sure half of your plate is filled with vegetables, at lunch and dinner.
- Choose wholegrain carbohydrates in moderation. So many people are 'carb-phobic' right now, but there is not strong enough evidence to really suggest we should avoid carbohydrates. In fact, they are a very important energy source. However, be smart about your choices – choose wholegrains that are high in fibre and aim to keep them to one-quarter of your plate, at lunch and dinner.
- Be sure to have lean protein choices at all your meals. Lean protein choices such as lean meat, fish, poultry, tofu and eggs will provide long-lasting energy when combined with carbohydrates at meals. Aim to have lean protein on one-quarter of your plate, at lunch and dinner.

**Do I need to count calories?**

NO! But that being said, at a very basic level, weight loss comes down to calories in and calories out. However, as with everything in life, it's not that simple. Despite what we have been led to believe, all calories are not created equally. Our body deals differently with the calories from refined carbohydrates (simple sugars) compared with the calories from fat and protein. Let's not get into the nitty-gritty of it, but understand that choosing high-fibre, low-sugar carbohydrates is just as important as watching total calorie intake. All of my recipes have been created with these theories in mind. So meals are nutrient-dense rather than calorie-dense. Rest assured, you don't need to take your calculator out and count calories – it has all been done for you right here!

Research also tells us that for weight loss people need to limit daily calorie intake to 1,200 and 1,500 calories per day for women and men, respectively. This is just a general guide and, remember, your activity level will also play a big role in your total calorie (energy) needs for the day. All my recipes have been analysed but to give you an idea, the average daily calorie intake on the two-week meal plan is 1,300 calories – well within normal ranges.

## IF I FOLLOW THESE RECOMMENDATIONS, WHAT CAN I EXPECT?

It is important to be realistic about your weight loss goals. Of course, most people want a magic wand that ensures whatever changes they make work within a week. Unfortunately that is not how long-term weight loss works.

In my experience a realistic target to aim for is 4–5 lbs of weight loss each month. Following this plan the longer term target would be 14 lbs (1 stone) every 3 months and 56 lbs (4 stone) over an entire year. The best news is that if you lose weight this way, you are more likely to keep it off. No point losing 2 stone in a month and gaining 3 stone back in the following few months, right?

Research demonstrates that losing 10% of weight when overweight/obese can help prevent and manage diseases and conditions such as type 2 diabetes, heart disease, raised cholesterol and raised blood pressure. Therefore, my recommendation is – if you are overweight/obese, set an initial weight loss target of 10% of your current weight. This may be less than your long-term target – but it is a realistic and achievable place to start. When you achieve that, you can set your next 10% weight loss target.

**Current weight (lbs) * 0.10 = _____ lbs of weight loss required**

## MOTIVATION TO MAKE A CHANGE: DO I NEED IT?

One of the most common questions I get asked when people come to me about making changes to their lifestyle is 'How do I keep motivated?' My answer often surprises people: 'You don't need it.' In part this is tongue-in-cheek, but I truly believe we rely too much on being highly motivated all the time. We should actually base our changes on things that take the lowest possible level of motivation, because for many of us this is actually the norm. And the research backs up my belief.

I was lucky enough to have been at a lecture given by B. J. Fogg[2] in California a few years back. The information he shared from his research changed everything I'd been saying to clients and shifted my focus on to how people can actually create permanent behaviour change in their lives. According to Fogg, motivation goes through peaks and troughs at different times of the day, week, year, and so on. You don't have to be a rocket scientist to know that, right? Fogg suggests that when motivation is high, it is a great time to make big changes that can have long-lasting effects on your week, month, year, and life. But what should we do when our motivation is low? This is when we need to focus on things that are easy to do. And rather than focusing on all the changes you want to make, we should actually focus on the triggers that make the healthy habits easy to do. I am going to repeat that so it really sticks: focus on the TRIGGERS that make the healthy habits EASY to do.

Let's take a look at some real-life examples.

I had a client, Tom, who was making some great changes in his life, but he found that his biggest downfall was when he went for coffee with his colleagues mid-afternoon. Tom was always tempted by the big cream cakes in the coffee shop and found it impossible to resist the temptation. This was really upsetting him, as he

---

2 B. J. Fogg is the director of the Persuasive Technology Lab at Stanford University. See *www.bjfogg.com*.

felt he was doing so well up until this point of the day. Unfortunately, this treat often triggered a downward spiral of high-fat, high-sugar foods. Tom wanted to know how he could increase his willpower and motivation to stop him giving in to this afternoon treat. At this point I wanted to focus more on the trigger – one that made it easy to only choose a cup of tea/coffee. The solution we came up with was that he would only bring enough money with him for his cup of tea/coffee. Tom felt this was the best solution for him because he didn't like to ask colleagues to lend him money and it limited his ability to buy the cake. This worked a treat for him!

Another client, Mary, was having trouble with exercise. She planned to exercise in the morning after dropping her children to school. But every morning was the same – chaos trying to get everyone in the house sorted. This led to Mary not planning much until she got back from the school run, by which point she just wanted to savour a cup of coffee and a biscuit and enjoy a quiet house. By the time she even thought about exercising it was too late. The simple trigger we incorporated into Mary's life was for her to have her workout gear left out from the night before and get dressed in it first thing in the morning. This simple change meant she was ready to exercise immediately after dropping the children to school and she still found time for her peaceful cup of tea at home afterwards. Win–win.

There are many triggers, but it is good to start thinking of the changes you want to make to your life, or your family's life, in this way. Whatever you do, remember to keep it simple! Focus on the triggers that make the healthy habits easy to do.

### Habits to help you live longer and better
Living longer and better is surely what we all strive for. Most people mistakenly believe that the road to achieve this is by dieting and exercising. I'm here to

let you in on a secret: they are wrong.[3] In fact, we see that people who incorporate just four habits into their lives will actually live longer and better **even if they are overweight** – surprised?

These habits are further confirmed when we look at studies done by Dan Buettner on areas around the world, known as 'blue zones', where people live the longest and with very little disease.[4] As mentioned above, we see some common traits in these areas in relation to eating and exercise habits:

1 Plant-based diet
2 Regular exercise/move naturally
3 No smoking
4 Alcohol in moderation

**The 80% rule: a rule to live by**
The 80% rule refers to the practice of learning to stop eating when your stomach feels 80% full. 'I don't even know what that feels like', I hear you shout! You are not alone. Most people go from starving to stuffed in a matter of minutes at mealtimes. This, unfortunately, is a consequence of bypassing your 'full' signals for years. The good news is that you CAN reconnect with it. Babies are born knowing innately when they are hungry and when they are full. They feed from their mother for as long as they need and they stop when they are full. However, as children get older, parents often encourage them to bypass this ability by forcing them to finish everything on their plate. By the time a person become an adult, they don't know what full really feels like any more, never mind 80% full.

Intuitive eating or mindful eating is a term given to the practice of being more connected with what and how much you are eating. I regularly run workshops in my

3  Matheson, E. M. *et al.* (2012), 'Healthy lifestyle habits and mortality in obese and over-weight individuals', *Journal of the American Board of Family Medicine*, vol. 25(1), 9–15.

4 Buettner, D. (2012), *The Blue Zones: 9 Lessons for Living Longer from the People Who've Lived the Longest.* Washington D. C.: National Geographic. See also *www.bluezones.com.*

# The Hunger Scale

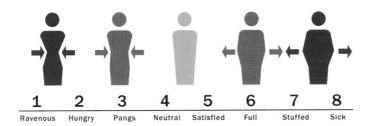

| 1 | 2 | 3 | 4 | 5 | 6 | 7 | 8 |
|---|---|---|---|---|---|---|---|
| Ravenous | Hungry | Pangs | Neutral | Satisfied | Full | Stuffed | Sick |

clinic for people who want to become more in tune with their 'hunger scale'.[5] This workshop is designed to help people listen to their body, savour their food and feel their best. The good news is that the workshop is easy and you can use it at any time. Here's how some of the steps work:

### Before eating: Pause to check in with your body
- Current hunger level: _____
- How full do you want to be when you finish eating? _____

### While eating: Savour and enjoy your food
- Focus on one bite at a time.
- Take small bites and chew thoroughly. Set down your fork and savour.
- Pause midway through the meal to assess your hunger: _____
- When you reach your desired fullness consider covering your meal or tidying up.

### After eating: Notice how you feel
- Fullness level immediately after the meal: _____
- Fullness level 20–30 minutes after eating: _____
- How do you feel? Do you feel satisfied and energised? Tired and sluggish?

5 https://fullplateliving.org/blog/it-hunger-or-it-cravings.

**Do you need rules to be healthy or to lose weight?**

I'm afraid there is no straight answer to this question; again, it's all in the approach. It is important to move away from a diet mentality and therefore important to reject diet rules. Remember, when your focus is on wellness (even when weight loss is part of that) there is no food list – no foods are off-limits; it is all about how much food you eat, and eating more intuitively. However, that being said, it is vital to look at what the research tells us about the habits people adopt who have been successful at losing weight and keeping it off.

The National Weight Control Registry[6] is following over 10,000 people in the United States who have lost significant amounts of weight and kept it off for long periods of time. The average weight loss has been 4 stone 10 lbs and average long-term weight loss spans 5.5 years. Most people in this study have the following habits in common; they:

- Eat breakfast
- Weigh themselves once/week
- Watch <10 hours of TV each week
- Exercise 1 hour each day.

I hope you can see a common theme appearing from the above research and from the other studies on the blue zones and living longer. It is about having sensible eating habits and exercising regularly.

Certain rules can actually work really well, but these rules need to come from YOU! The rules you make need to resonate with your soul; they need to be ones that YOU feel strongly about – this will make them easier to follow and they won't require high levels of motivation.

---

6 The National Weight Control Registry was established in 1994 by Rena Wing, PhD, from Brown Medical School, Rhode Island, and James O. Hill, PhD, from the University of Colorado. See *www.nwcr.ws*.

Here are some real-life examples of personal 'rules' that work for people. I'll include myself here and let you in on a little secret of mine … I am a chocoholic, so I need to have certain 'rules' in my life to manage how much of it I eat. One rule that has worked great for me is: no chocolate, or other treats, before 12 noon. This one makes sense to me, because I feel anything before noon is breakfast food and I don't consider chocolate breakfast food.

Another client of mine, Annie, was having difficulty managing the volume of wine she was drinking. She didn't have an alcohol dependency issue, but she noticed that when she opened a bottle of wine on a Friday night, invariably she finished it. This was an area she really wanted to change as it was having a negative effect on her healthy living attempts. It led to eating more junk on a Friday night and limited exercise on a Saturday morning. The rule she felt worked best for her was to buy a half bottle of wine and to only keep one in the house at any one time. This worked well as it limited the volume Annie drank, but she still got to enjoy her wine on a Friday night, and it didn't interfere with her other healthy living goals.

As long as the 'rules' you set are healthy and sensible, I think they can work really well with some basic healthy living habits I recommend for people.

**Healthy living habits**
- Eat regular meals and snacks – aim to eat every 3 hours.
- Follow your hunger and fullness signals – stop eating when you are 80% full.
- Make sure to get your 5-a-day of fruits and vegetables, as a minimum.
- Drink water regularly – aim for 2 litres a day.
- Make exercise a part of your daily life.

**No foods are off-limits? Really?**

This is often something people find very difficult to get their heads around. The most common experience when following a 'diet' is that there are certain foods that you must avoid. However, when you take a different approach and you are eating for wellness, no foods are off-limits. Of course, ultimately it comes down to the volume of food you eat. So, even if you have a very rich meal and you stop eating when you are 80% full, it can still fit into your healthy living plan. I have to be honest, it is more difficult to train yourself to do this, but the rewards will stick with you for life and not just a few weeks.

## LET'S TALK ABOUT FOOD

At a very basic level, the function of food is to provide energy. Food in the twenty-first century has become so much more than just energy – in most cultures around the world, it is a big part of social gatherings too. This is not a problem as long as you enjoy and savour the food you eat and stop eating when you are 80% full. As you make these recipes, make sure that you enjoy the taste, flavour and texture of each meal – it is time to really start savouring the food you eat.

I am always asked about foods that boost energy, so let's look at that.

**Nutrition basics**

NUTRIENT: Carbohydrate
FOUND IN: Bread, potatoes, rice, pasta, cereal, fruit, fruit juice and milk
BEST CHOICES: Wholegrains, e.g. brown instead of white for starches
BENEFITS: Long-lasting energy

NUTRIENT: Protein
FOUND IN: Lean meat, fish, poultry, eggs, nuts, dairy, beans, legumes
BEST CHOICES: Lean sources that are baked/grilled and without skin
BENEFITS: Provides long-lasting energy when teamed with high-fibre carbohydrates

NUTRIENT: Fat
FOUND IN: Fried foods, fish, meat, nuts, seeds, dairy
BEST CHOICES: Fish and plant-based sources = unsaturated sources
BENEFITS: Unsaturated sources = immune-boosting properties

### Label reading

In an ideal world, we would only eat food we make ourselves and never eat packaged food. But in the real world, this isn't always feasible. Sometimes there is too much focus on only eating the 'perfect' food when sometimes the 'good enough' food can keep you on the straight and narrow when life gets crazy.

When choosing packaged foods, you should aim for foods that are low in fat, in particular saturated fat, low in sugar and high in fibre. Here are the numbers you should be looking for to reach those goals.

**Guideline amounts per 100g**

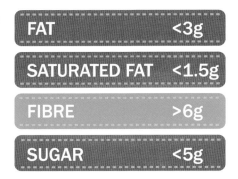

| FAT | <3g |
| SATURATED FAT | <1.5g |
| FIBRE | >6g |
| SUGAR | <5g |

### How to set yourself up for success

It is all about managing your environment and there are two key places that you need to give some special attention to. The first at home; the second is the supermarket. Unfortunately, in the supermarket you are not in control of where products are placed and other marketing strategies that entice you to buy certain foods. However, in your own home you are in complete control. You need to grab that control with both hands and set yourself up for success with a well-planned kitchen.

### A well-planned kitchen

**OUT OF SIGHT, OUT OF MIND:** Keep treats that tempt you out of the house. You don't have to be a martyr to the cause of living well – make it easy on yourself and avoid bringing foods that trigger unhealthy food choices into the home.

**MAKE THE HEALTHY CHOICE EASY:** Whether you are trying to drink more water or eat more fruit, think about what will make those goals easier to do. Leave a jug of water on the counter when you are at home so that you can sip away throughout the day, or have fruit you enjoy washed and ready to eat and visible on the counter, to achieve your goal – don't hide away the healthy choices. Make sure vegetables are at eye level in the fridge to ensure these are the foods that greet you every time you open the fridge.

**PLAN AHEAD:** Make time each week to peel and chop vegetables, and then place them in airtight bags or containers in the fridge so that they are easy to access for dinners and/or snacks. A regular theme that has come up for *Operation Transformation* leaders is a complete lack of planning, which makes this tip essential. My tip is to use Sunday of each week to plan the week ahead. You will be surprised by how much a positive impact spending 1–2 hours on a Sunday getting organised can make to your week.

**PLANNING PERMISSION:** Just like when you are looking to extend your house and you need to apply for planning permission, you should think about what foods you are going to allow into your house and where you're going to store them, especially if treats need to be kept in the home for an occasion such as Christmas or a birthday party. I recommend picking a press that you don't use that often, or placing them at the back of a press, so that you don't see them a lot. The biggest mistake people make is to put them in a press that they need to open regularly and before they know it, they are back in the supermarket buying all the same food again, originally bought for that special occasion!

### Pantry basics

Be sure to have the following basics in your cupboards to make it easier to rustle up some of these meals with short notice.

**BASICS:** Rapeseed oil (for foods cooked at high temperatures), olive oil (for warm foods or foods at cold/room temperature), salt, pepper and peppercorns, reduced-sodium vegetable stock, reduced-sodium chicken stock, reduced-sodium beef stock, butter, plain flour, breadcrumbs (keep in freezer), cornflour, dark brown sugar, mayonnaise, ketchup

**CARBOHYDRATES:** Wholegrain rice, couscous, quinoa, wholewheat pasta, wholewheat noodles, polenta, potatoes

**SPICES:** Chilli powder, dried oregano, paprika, smoked paprika, cumin, dried coriander, five-spice powder, dried basil, rosemary, sage, dill, desiccated coconut, thyme, crushed red pepper, cocoa powder, mustard powder

**JARS:** Sun-dried tomato pesto, basil pesto (as back-up, fresh is best), curry paste (from a speciality shop), Worcestershire sauce, easy ginger, easy garlic (as a back-up), hot sauce, orange marmalade, mango chutney, wholegrain mustard, Dijon mustard, balsamic vinegar, honey, sweet chilli sauce, rice vinegar, reduced-sodium soy sauce, teriyaki sauce, cider vinegar, salsa, fish sauce

**CANS:** Chopped tomatoes, tomato purée, sweetcorn, tuna in spring water, kidney beans, black beans, light coconut milk, chickpeas, bamboo shoots

### Supermarket tips

Limiting time spent in the supermarket and using your time there effectively is important. So many people have the best of intentions but as soon as they enter the supermarket everything seems to go wrong. 'Why does this happen?' people ask me regularly. There are many reasons, but one thing that we have to be very clear about is that the supermarket's goal is to make you buy more. They employ consumer shopper behaviourists, psychologists and other experts to figure out how this can happen. They aim to engage all your senses to entice you to buy more than you planned.

Unfortunately, many of the foods that are marketed aggressively are of the unhealthy variety, but there are some interesting studies out there on what happens when these experts employ the same tactics for healthy foods. Researchers at New Mexico State University looked at the impact of partitioning a shopping trolley.[7] Half of the shopping trolley was separated with a card that instructed shoppers to place their fruit and vegetables in front of the card. This simple strategy doubled the amount of fruit and vegetables purchased by customers in this supermarket.

When it comes to food shopping, people don't buy rationally. So many things, from your emotional state to your energy levels, can affect what you buy. But there are practices you can put in place to protect yourself against all this and to ensure you leave the supermarket with the foods that are going to nourish you and your family.

**Setting yourself up for success in the supermarket**
- Being organised and prepared is essential – this starts at home!
- Pick a time in the week to plan your meals for the week ahead.
- Check your cupboards and make a list to ensure you have all the ingredients you need. Make sure you are not hungry or tired when making this list.
- Go to the supermarket with the list in hand. Make sure you are NOT hungry, tired, emotional, angry, annoyed, bored or lonely – granted, it can be hard to achieve this!
- Be aware of the tactics supermarkets employ to make you buy more. Remember, you are not saving money if you go for a 'buy 2 get 1 free' offer if you

7 Wansink, B. *et al.* (2014), 'Partitioned shopping carts: assortment allocation cues that increase fruit and vegetable purchases'. See *http://ssrn.com/abstract=2473647* or *http://dx.doi. org/10.2139/ssrn.2473647.*

never intended to buy the product in the first place.
- Stick to your list.
- Aim to fill one-third of your basket or trolley with fruit and vegetables.
- Avoid the aisles that have treats which tempt you. Manage your environment!

## CAN I DRINK ALCOHOL?

A very simple rule of thumb is 'the less alcohol you drink, the more weight you lose'. That being said, moderate amounts of alcohol for adults is not a problem. However, it is essential to have alcohol-free days in your week. The low-risk guideline for men is $\leq 17$ units each week and for women $\leq 11$ units each week. These units should be spread out over the week with no more than 6 units in one sitting. A unit = half pint stout/lager/cider, 100 ml glass of wine, a pub measure of spirits. However, these recommendations are not for weight loss. Therefore, I would recommend limiting alcohol as much as possible, ideally to just once a week or 2–3 units.

## TIPS TO AVOID COMMON PITFALLS

**MAKE SURE TO EAT REGULARLY:** Often people think the less they eat, the more weight they will lose, and will often cut out snacks. However, eating little and often is essential to keep your metabolism moving and burning. Therefore, having three meals and two snacks each and every day is really important.

**WEIGH YOUR PORTIONS:** None of us have the magical ability to estimate portions accurately. From my 10 years' experience in private practice and particularly my experience on *Operation Transformation* I have seen this belief undermine weight loss attempts. When you are making changes at the start, it is essential to use a weighing scales to accurately measure portion sizes. As time goes on, you can compare the weighed portion with your own household serving spoons and use these for the long term.

**EATING OUT:** The good news is that you do not have to avoid eating out. I am a strong believer in making changes

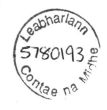

that you can live with for life and it would be unrealistic to think you are never going to eat out again. Eating out can and should be a very enjoyable experience, and it is important to be able to enjoy the social occasions that go along with eating out, without worrying that you have blown all your healthy eating plans. However, eating out too often is not going to help you lose weight – limit it to once a week at most. Here are some tips when eating out:

1 Plan ahead. If the menu is available online, it can really help to have a look at it and flag a few meals that you think will work for you. That way, even if you get distracted when ordering, you will already have your prep work done.
2 Don't arrive at the restaurant hungry, as you will be much more tempted to devour the bread basket! Make sure to have a small snack about an hour before leaving your house.
3 Order food your way. For example, ask for extra vegetables or a salad instead of chips, if these are recommendations you want to stick to.
4 Stop eating when you are 80% full. You don't have to finish everything on your plate. When you feel 80% full, place your napkin over your remaining food so you are less likely to go back to it.
5 Share a dessert! If you feel like dessert, go for it. But suggest sharing it with someone else and really savour every bite.

**I've fallen off the wagon, now what?**
No matter how bad a meal, a day, a weekend or a holiday has been, the sooner you get back on track the better. Remember, no one meal can undo all the good work of an entire week. The most common mistake is to keep eating with the idea that 'I've ruined it now, I'll start again tomorrow'. But this is really a diet mentality and something that it is best to get out of. It might mean going for an extra walk in the week or making your next meal lighter, but either way just get back on track as soon as you can.

Holidays can generally put a spanner in the works. First and foremost, you have to enjoy holiday time, but do remember, nothing adds to post-holiday blues like an extra half a stone! Don't forget the main goal during holidays is to maintain weight – you shouldn't be trying to actively lose weight. The difficult thing on holidays is that you may be eating out for most of your meals and you don't really have control over how your meals are prepared. Here are some tips to keep you in balance so that you enjoy your holiday and maintain your weight:

# WHAT HAPPENS WHEN I GO ON HOLIDAYS?

1 You are not on a diet. The only goal is to maintain your weight.
2 Keep your routine. Don't skip meals, especially breakfast – aim to have three meals and two snacks daily. Keep one of your midday meals a little lighter if your evening meal is the main event!
3 Eat intuitively. Continue to be conscious of what you are eating and how full you are feeling. Stop eating when you are 80% full. You will actually enjoy your meals more.
5 Drink water regularly. It can be tempting to drink sugar-sweetened drinks in hot weather, but try to stick to water with lemon and/or lime to limit unnecessary calories.
6 KEEP MOVING. If you do nothing else, just make sure to keep moving; that may be walking, swimming, cycling. Whatever it is, aim to have at least 30 minutes of moderately intense exercise each day.

# A LITTLE BIT ABOUT THE RECIPES

The recipes I have chosen are my favourites from my last few years on *Operation Transformation*. All of the recipes are designed for an adult who is trying to make healthy changes to their lifestyle and to lose weight. The recipes are set up so that 1/2 of your plate is vegetables, 1/4 protein and 1/4 carbohydrate (see illustration). Most importantly, though, all the recipes are designed to taste good!

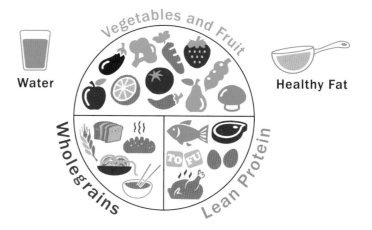

## WHERE ARE THE DESSERT RECIPES?

In case you haven't noticed yet, I hate to break it to you but there are no dessert recipes. The main reason for this is that while I love to bake, it is not my forte and coming up with 'healthy' dessert recipes really isn't my thing! Instead, I would much prefer to see you enjoy a treat – whatever that may be – but try not to do it too often. Desserts are something to be savoured, and when kept to special occasions I think they are something that can be enjoyed as part of a healthy, balanced eating plan.

Enjoy!

# WEEKLY PLANS

Being organised and prepared is half the battle when trying to make changes to your lifestyle and eating habits. So to help get you started, I have come up with some sample weekly plans that you can work off until you get the hang of it yourself. None of this is set in stone, so if you wish, change any of the options here to another recipe that can work too. Enjoy!

# WEEK 1

| MEAL | MONDAY | TUESDAY | WEDNESDAY | THURSDAY | FRIDAY | SATURDAY | SUNDAY |
|------|--------|---------|-----------|----------|--------|----------|--------|
| BREAKFAST | Overnight Oats | Boiled Egg and English Muffin | Porridge and Raspberries | Breakfast Sandwich | Porridge and Banana | Mini Grill | Tropical Muesli Cup |
| SNACK | Fruit and Nuts: 1 medium apple and 6 almonds | Fruit and Nuts: 1 small banana and 6 almonds | Fruit and Nuts: 1 small banana and 2 brazil nuts | Beetroot and Orange Smoothie Shot | Fruit Cup | Crackers and Cheese | Baked Berry Square |
| LUNCH | Wholemeal Hot Chicken Pitta Pocket | Sunshine Salad | Tuna Panzanella Salad | Cup of Soup and Open Tuna Sandwich | Toasted Special | BBQ Chicken Salad | Herby Roast Chicken |
| SNACK | Veggies and Hummus: 1 stick of celery and 1 tbsp hummus | Fruit and Nuts: 1 medium orange and 6 almonds | Veggies and Hummus: 1/2 red pepper and 1 tbsp hummus | Beetroot and Orange Smoothie | Baked Berry Square | Fruit Cup | Smoked Salmon Roll |
| DINNER | Spaghetti Bolognese | Turkey Pesto Pasta | Curry Beef Noodle Bowl | Spanish Chicken | Sea Bass with Salsa-Inspired Sauce | Cheeseburger and Fries | Caprese Pasta Salad |

# WEEK 2

| MEAL | MONDAY | TUESDAY | WEDNESDAY | THURSDAY | FRIDAY | SATURDAY | SUNDAY |
|------|--------|---------|-----------|----------|--------|----------|--------|
| BREAKFAST | Overnight Oats | Berry and Chia Smoothie | Overnight Oats | Breakfast Sandwich | Cereal with Fruit | French Toast | Hot Start |
| SNACK | Fruit Cup | Fruit and Nuts: 1 small banana and 6 almonds | Spinach and Mango Smoothie | Fruit and Nuts: 1 medium orange and 6 almonds | Baked Berry Square | Fruit and Nuts: 1 medium apple and 1 tsp peanut butter | Baked Berry Square |
| LUNCH | Tantalising Tuna Salad | Chicken and Lentil Hot Bowl | Turkey Club Sandwich | Cup of Soup and Open Ham Sandwich | Spinach Salad with Chicken, Corn and Feta | Chicken Noodle Soup | Chicken and Loaded-Vegetable Bake |
| SNACK | Baked Berry Square | Crackers and Cheese | Spinach and Mango Smoothie | Fruit and Nuts: 1 medium apple and 1 tsp peanut butter | Fruit Cup | Smoked Salmon Roll | Veggies and Hummus: 1 stick of celery and 1 tbsp hummus |
| DINNER | Chicken Fajitas | Creamy Mushroom Pasta | Beef and Rice | Granny Brid's Chicken | Mexican Cod | Italian Steak | Open Salmon and Dill Mayo Sandwich |

# WEEK 3

| MEAL | MONDAY | TUESDAY | WEDNESDAY | THURSDAY | FRIDAY | SATURDAY | SUNDAY |
|------|--------|---------|-----------|----------|--------|----------|--------|
| BREAKFAST | Berry and Chia Smoothie | Porridge and Raspberries | Breakfast Sandwich | Porridge and Strawberries | Berry and Chia Smoothie | Mini Grill | Mediterranean Breakfast Pitta |
| SNACK | Fruit Cup | Baked Berry Square | Fruit and Nuts: 1 medium orange and 6 almonds | Veggies and Hummus: 1 stick of celery and 1 tbsp hummus | Crackers and Cheese | Baked Berry Square | Fruit Cup |
| LUNCH | BBQ Chicken Salad | Chicken Noodle Soup | Baked Ham and Cheese Sandwich | Cup of Soup and Open Smoked Salmon Sandwich | Chicken Salad Sandwich | Baked Tomato with Goat's Cheese | Lasagne and Salad |
| SNACK | Veggies and Hummus: 1 carrot and 1 tbsp hummus | Fruit and Nuts: 1 medium banana and 6 almonds | Spinach and Mango Smoothie | Fruit Cup | Fruit and Nuts: 1 medium apple and 6 almonds | Fruit and Nuts: 1 medium banana and 6 almonds | Beetroot and Orange Smoothie |
| DINNER | Fish Cakes and Salad | Spicy Pork and Carrot Stir-Fry | Mango Chicken | Goat's Cheese and Beetroot Salad | Quick Fish Stew | Thai Red Curry and Fried Rice | Hearty Chickpea Soup |

# WEEK 4

| MEAL | MONDAY | TUESDAY | WEDNESDAY | THURSDAY | FRIDAY | SATURDAY | SUNDAY |
|---|---|---|---|---|---|---|---|
| BREAKFAST | Porridge and Blueberries | Boiled Egg and English Muffin | Overnight Oats | Breakfast Sandwich | Porridge and Banana | Cinnamon and Yogurt Pancakes | Mushroom and Ricotta Omelette |
| SNACK | Beetroot and Orange Smoothie | Baked Berry Square | Fruit Cup | Fruit and Nuts: 1 medium apple and 2 brazil nuts | Fruit and Nuts: 1 medium orange and 6 almonds | Fruit and Nuts: 1 medium orange and 2 brazil nuts | Fruit Cup |
| LUNCH | Cup of Soup and Open Tuna Sandwich | Spinach Salad with Chicken, Corn and Feta | Baked Ham and Cheese Sandwich | Tempting Turkey Salad and Crisp Bread | Chicken Salad Pitta | Chicken Noodle Soup | Roast Basil Chicken |
| SNACK | Cheese and Crackers | Fruit and Nuts: 1 medium apple and 2 brazil nuts | Cheese and Crackers | Veggies and Hummus: red pepper and 1 tbsp hummus | Baked Berry Square | Cheese and Crackers | Baked Berry Square |
| DINNER | Meatballs and Spaghetti | Chicken Parmesan | Sweet and Sour Pork | Chicken Goujons | Teriyaki Salmon and Coriander Rice | Saturday Night Pizza Special | Cup of Soup and Open Smoked Salmon Sandwich |

BREAKFAST REALLY IS THE MOST IMPORTANT MEAL OF THE DAY. I RECOMMEND THAT YOU EAT SOMETHING WITHIN AN HOUR OF GETTING UP IN THE MORNING. NO MATTER WHERE I AM OR WHAT I'M DOING, I ALWAYS MAKE SURE TO START MY DAY WITH BREAKFAST.

BREA

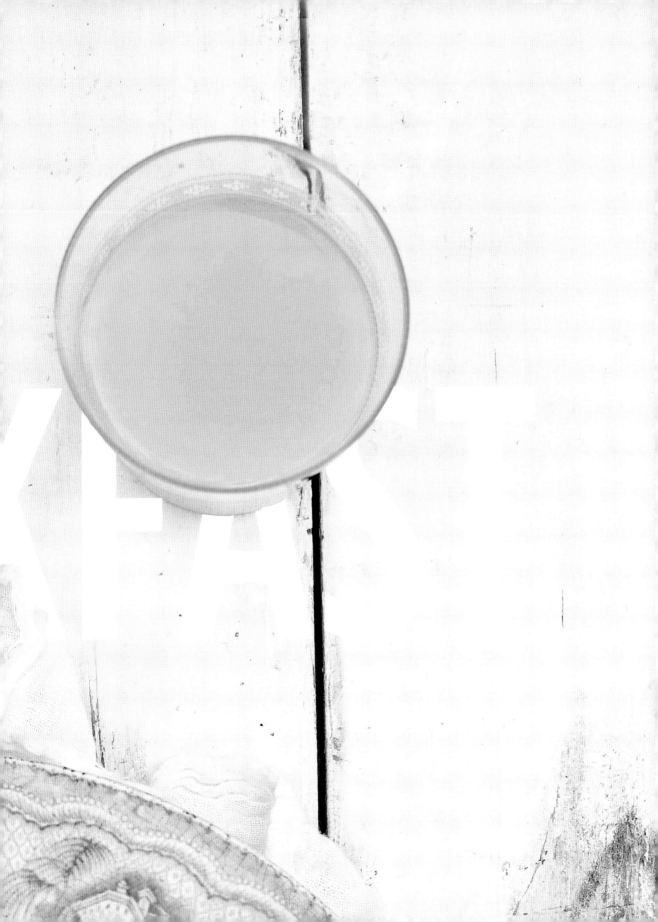

# QUICK AND EASY BREAKFASTS
# PORRIDGE AND FRUIT

A winter warmer – porridge is a staple in my home. You can mix it up with different fruit for variety.

## Serves 1

30 g oats
150 ml low-fat milk
1 tsp cinnamon
½ tsp nutmeg
1 tsp honey

FRUIT OPTIONS:
1 small banana
90 g strawberries
90 g raspberries
90 g blueberries
20 g raisins

## Calories:
Porridge 219
Porridge and banana 276
Porridge and strawberries 255
Porridge and raspberries 257
Porridge and blueberries 259
Porridge and raisins 278

› Place the oats with the low-fat milk and cook for 90 seconds in the microwave or 3–5 minutes on the stove top.
› Sprinkle with cinnamon and nutmeg.
› Top with sliced fruit and honey.
› Serve hot.

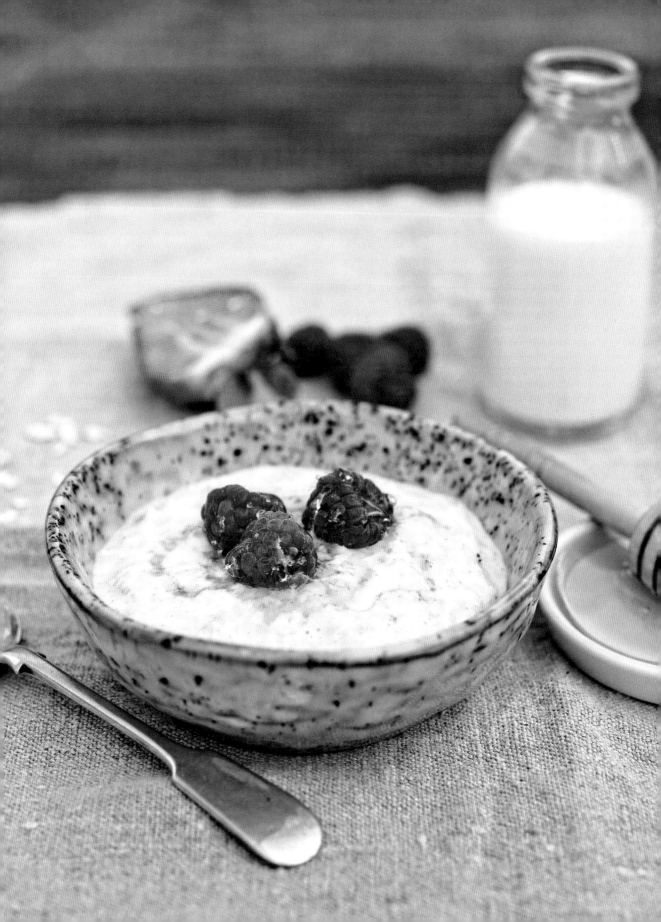

# BOILED EGG AND ENGLISH MUFFIN

*A quick way to get eggs in mid-week.* **Serves 1**

1 egg
1 wholemeal English muffin
1 tsp butter

**Calories:**
243

› Place the egg in a pot of boiling water and boil for 3–6 minutes. Once cooked, remove from the pot carefully. Allow the egg to cool and then peel and slice.
› Place the muffin in the toaster and toast as desired.
› Carefully remove the toasted muffin from the toaster and, when cooled, spread with butter.
› Place the sliced boiled egg on top of the muffin.

# OVERNIGHT OATS

› Mix all the ingredients in a bowl or Tupperware container.
› Cover with clingfilm or a lid.
› Refrigerate for at least 3 hours or overnight to soften the oats.
› Store up to 6 days or freeze in containers for later consumption. Thaw frozen containers in the refrigerator overnight or in the microwave for 1–2 minutes.

I love, love this recipe. Another great winter warmer and so handy when made ahead of time. **Serves 2**

45 g rolled oats (or pinhead oats)
120 ml low-fat milk
60 g natural yogurt (3% fat)
70 g mixed berries or preferred fruit (fresh or frozen)
1 tbsp chia seeds, milled flaxseed or chopped nuts
pinch of cinnamon
$1/4$ tsp vanilla extract
2 tsp honey

**Calories:**
193

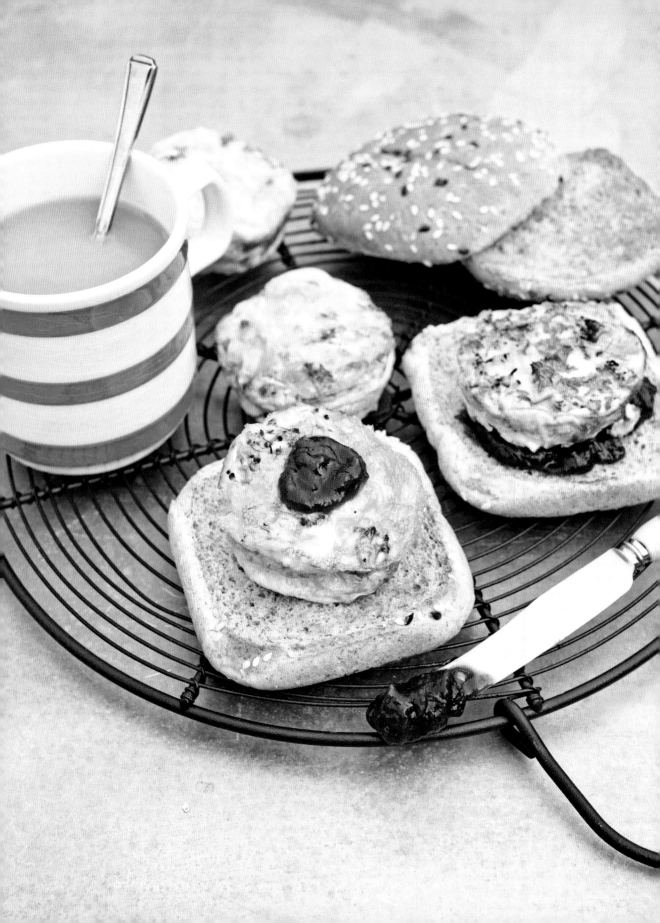

# BREAKFAST SANDWICH

› Preheat the oven to 200°C/400°F/gas 6 and prepare a muffin tin. Spraying non-stick spray on paper liners will allow for easier removal.
› Cook the chopped broccoli (or other vegetables) by steaming or sautéing for about 5 minutes. Prep the ingredients while the broccoli cooks.
› In a medium bowl, crack and whisk the eggs. Add the milk, mustard, salt, pepper, spring onion and parsley. Whisk again.
› Add the grated cheese to the egg mixture.
› When the broccoli is cooked, divide equally among the muffin cups. Then pour the egg mixture evenly into the muffin cups.
› Place in the oven for 18–22 minutes, or until the eggs set (when the top becomes light golden and/or a toothpick comes out clean).
› Place in a large Baggie or container to refrigerate or freeze until ready to eat. You can reheat straight from the freezer in the microwave for 30–60 seconds.
› To serve, toast the halved English muffin, or bun, until lightly golden. Spread the relish evenly over the slices. Place the quiche on one half and top with the other.

This recipe is great to cook ahead and freeze in individual portions. A great option for children of all ages as well. As this is a cook-ahead breakfast, I would recommend that you cook all six servings and freeze the extra portions. **Serves 6 (1 cup per serving)**

90 g broccoli or other vegetables (fresh or frozen), chopped
3 eggs
70 ml low-fat milk
$1/4$ tsp mustard powder
pinch of salt and pepper (optional)
1 spring onion, chopped
1 tbsp chopped parsley
30 g Cheddar cheese, grated
6 wholemeal English muffins/ wholemeal buns (40 g) (1 per serving)
2 tsp tomato relish per serving

**Calories:**
217

# BERRY AND CHIA SMOOTHIE

A great recipe when you are on the go and you need to bring something with you! **Serves 1**

125g frozen berries
10 g spinach
2 small carrots
1 fresh mandarin or 70 g tinned in own juice
90 ml almond milk
60 g natural yogurt (3% fat)
2 tsp chia seeds

**Calories:**
199

› Boil the frozen berries. Then blend all ingredients until smooth.

# WEEKEND BREAKFAST TREATS
## HOT START

I find it's nice to change things up a little at the weekend. These breakfast recipes are a little higher in calories, so I suggest you enjoy them just once a week.

› Prep the tomatoes and mushrooms.
› Heat the oil and gently fry the egg over a medium heat.
› Lightly fry the tomatoes and mushrooms.
› Toast and butter the bread and top with the fried egg, tomatoes and mushrooms.

Nice for a treat at the weekend!
**Serves 1**

1 tomato, chopped
50g mushrooms, chopped
1 egg
$^1/_2$ tbsp olive oil
1 slice wholemeal bread
1 tsp butter

**Calories**
284

# CONTINENTAL FRUIT SALAD

A fresh summertime option – but can be made at any time of the year using fruit that's in season.

**Serves 1**

240 g fresh fruit salad (kiwis, peaches, passionfruit)
30 g natural yogurt (3% fat)
1 tbsp honey
1 tsp milled flaxseed or linseed

**Calories:**
282

› Chop the fruit and place in a bowl.
› Top with natural yogurt, honey and flaxseed or linseed.

# OMELETTE

› Mix the eggs and milk in a bowl, and set aside.
› Choose one of the filler options below and chop the vegetable(s).
› Add a pinch of salt and pepper to the eggs.
› Heat the oil in a pan at a medium heat.
› Add the desired filler to the egg mixture.
› Pour into the pan and allow the egg mixture to cook around the edges.
› Lift up one side of the omelette to check if the egg has slightly browned. The middle part of the mixture will still be a bit runny.
› Once the bottom is browned, you can either turn it over to cook, or place under the grill (on medium heat) for 5–7 minutes, until browned on top and the inside is completely cooked and no longer runny.

### Calories:
Mushroom and ricotta omelette 305
Mixed pepper omelette 344
Goat's cheese and spinach omelette 316
Bacon and tomato omelette 330

A nice change from cereal, and eggs are a great protein option for breakfast. **Serves 1**

2 eggs
25 ml low-fat milk
pinch of salt and pepper
1 tsp rapeseed oil

FILLER OPTIONS:
**Mushroom and Ricotta**
100 g mushrooms, chopped
25 g ricotta cheese

**Mixed Pepper**
$1/2$ red pepper, deseeded and chopped
$1/2$ yellow pepper, deseeded and chopped
20 g ricotta cheese
1 tomato, chopped

**Goat's Cheese and Spinach**
30 g goat's cheese
100 g spinach

**Bacon and Tomato**
50 g cooked rashers, grilled and chopped
1 tomato, chopped

# MINI GRILL

A modified 'full Irish' which hits the spot for a change at the weekend.

**Serves 1**

1 tsp olive oil
1 egg
2 turkey rashers
100 g baked beans
160 ml orange juice

**Calories:**
274

› Heat the oil and gently fry the egg over a medium heat.
› Place the rashers under the grill.
› Heat the beans.
› When cooked, place all on a plate to serve.

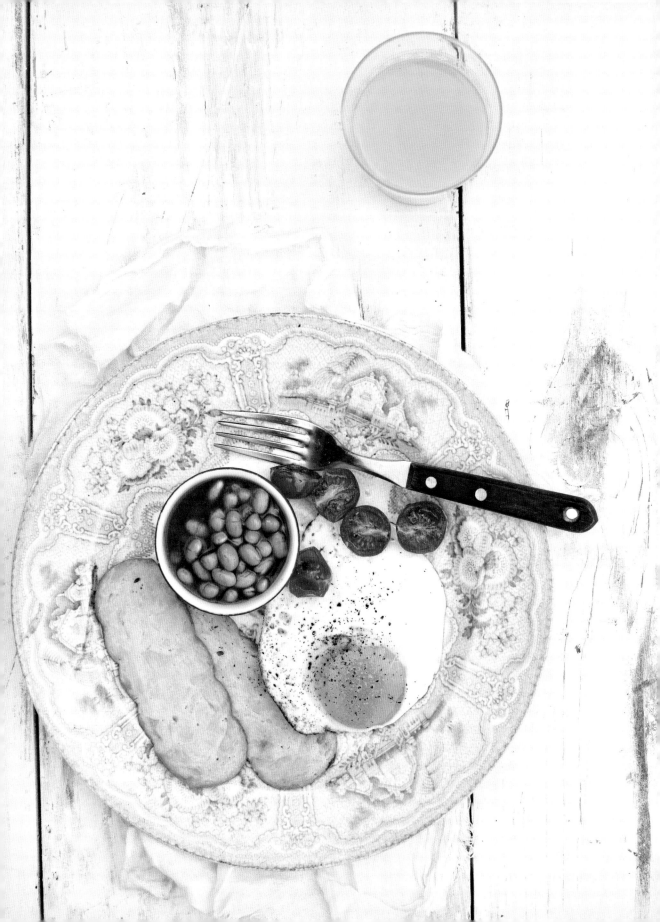

# TROPICAL MUESLI CUP

Have chopped fruit at the ready to be able to make this fresh breakfast quickly at the weekend

**Serves 2**

15 g oats
$^1/_2$ tbsp almonds, chopped
1 tbsp granola with raisins
40 ml boiled water, slightly cooled
1 kiwi, peeled and chopped
150 g pineapple, peeled and
    chopped
30 g natural yogurt (3% fat)
$^1/_2$ tbsp honey

**Calories:**
349

› Combine the oats, almonds and granola in a bowl.
› Add the water and set aside to soak for
  10– 15 minutes.
› Divide into two bowls, layer with fruit and top with
  natural yogurt and honey.

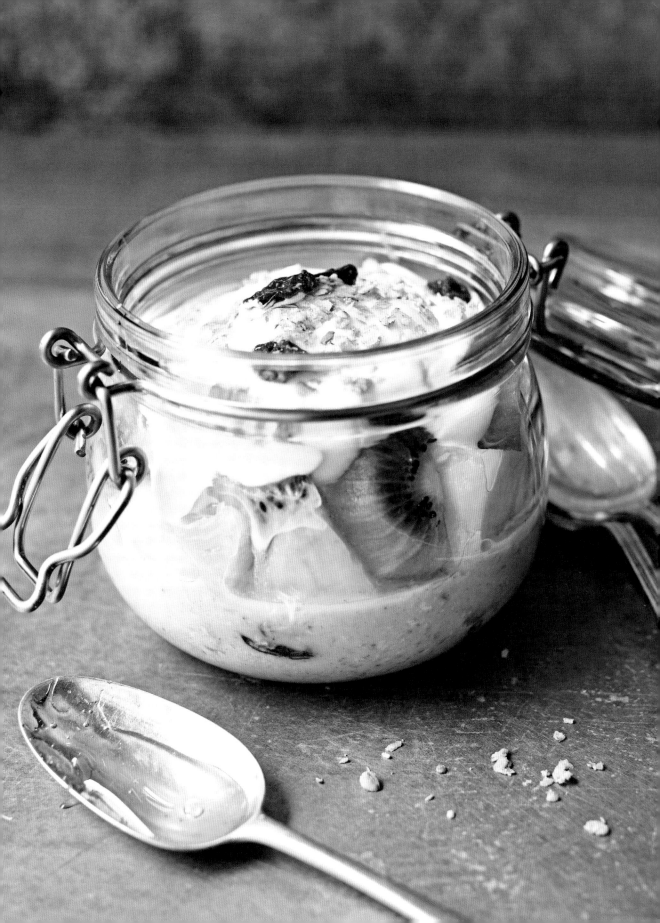

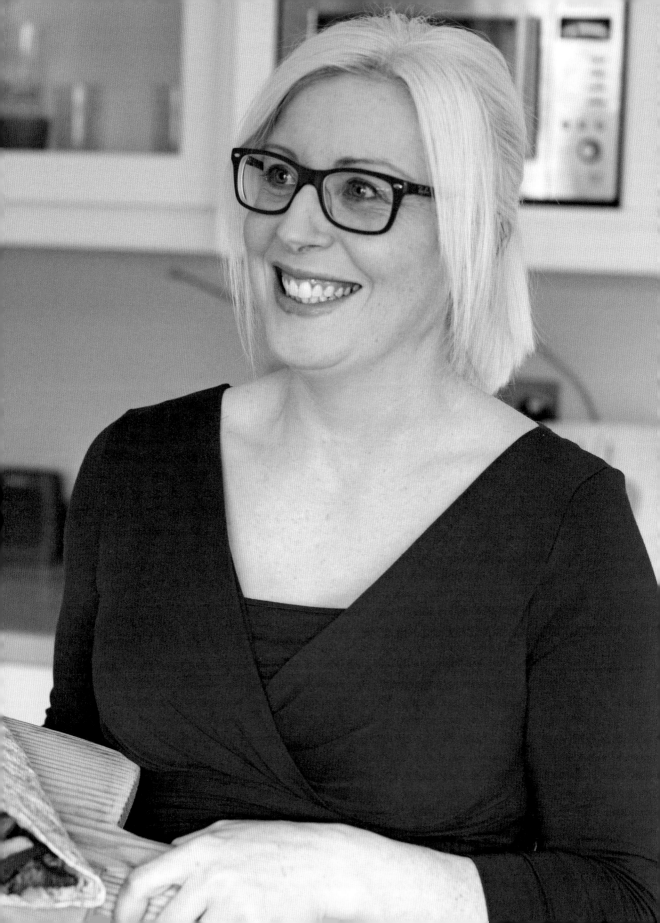

# MEDITERRANEAN BREAKFAST PITTA

> Place the egg in a pot of boiling water and boil for 3–6 minutes. Once cooked, remove from pot carefully. Allow the egg to cool and then peel and slice.
> Place the pitta in the toaster and toast as desired.
> Carefully remove from the toaster when done and slice open when cool – pitta may be hot, so be careful doing this.
> Spread light cream cheese in the pitta and layer with the spinach, tomato and boiled egg.

Store cooked boiled eggs in the fridge to make this a quick option.
**Serves 1**

1 egg
1 wholemeal round pitta
30 g light cream cheese
30 g spinach
1 tomato, sliced

**Calories:**
379

# CINNAMON AND YOGURT PANCAKES

Who doesn't love pancakes? A great option for kids at the weekend.

**Serves 2**

125 g self-raising flour
15 g caster sugar
1 tsp cinnamon
120 g natural yogurt (3% fat)
1 egg, beaten
6 tbsp low-fat milk
2 tsp butter
2 tsp honey
70 g fruit

**Calories:**
389

› Put the flour in a mixing bowl with the sugar and cinnamon. In a separate bowl, mix 100 g of the yogurt, beaten egg and milk with a fork.
› Make a well in the middle of the dry mixture and then add the wet mixture. (You can add more milk if the batter is too thick.)
› Place a pan on a medium heat and add 1 teaspoon of butter.
› Pour half of the mixture into the pan, turning when brown on one side.
› When cooked – the pancake will be light and fluffy and not very thin – remove from the pan.
› Top each pancake with the remaining natural yogurt (10 g per pancake), 1 teaspoon of honey and 35 g of fruit.

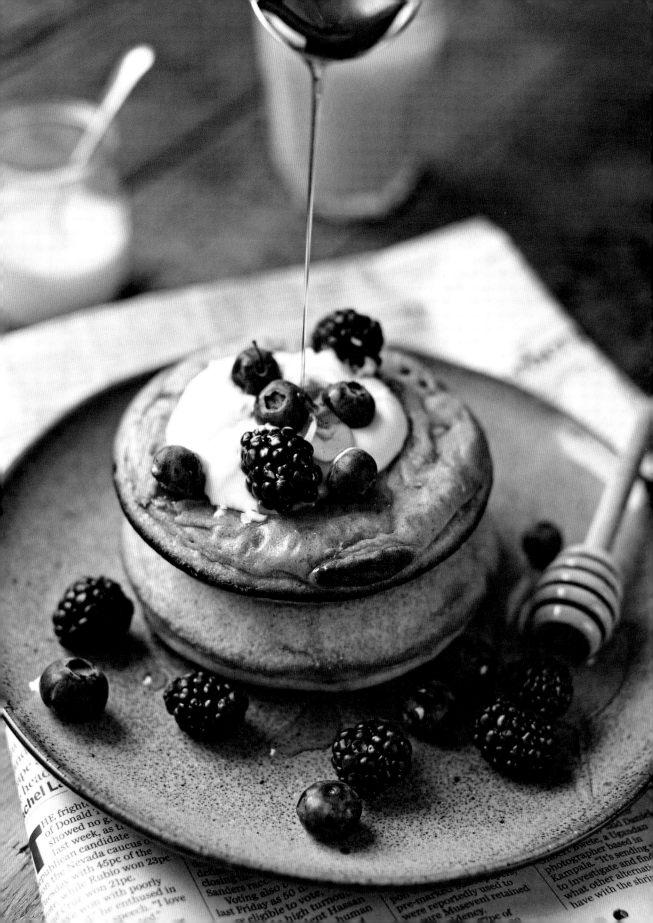

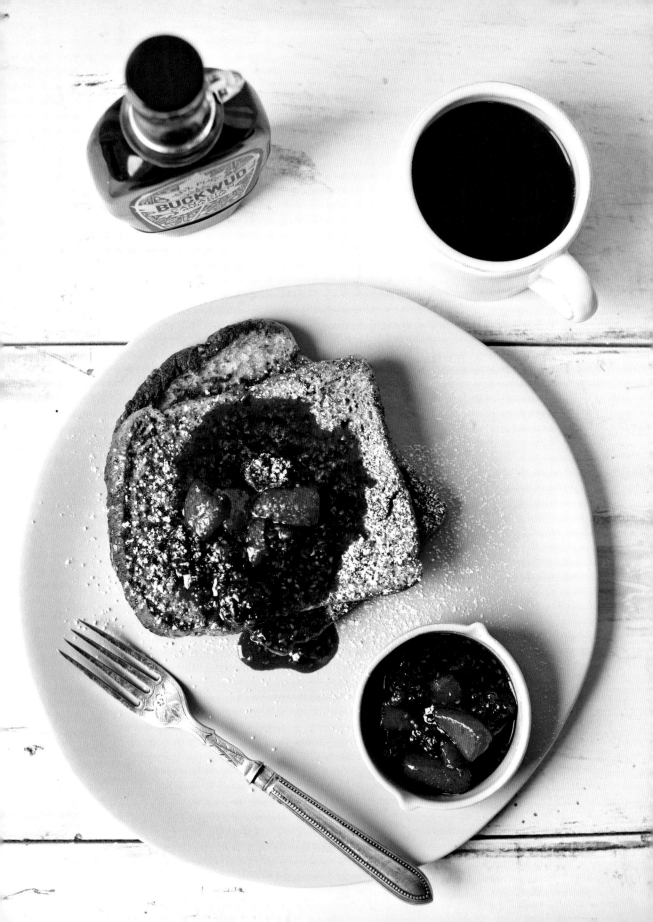

# FRENCH TOAST

- › In a bowl, mix the egg, milk and cinnamon.
- › Melt the butter in a frying pan until softened.
- › Dip the bread in the egg mixture, soaking each side well.
- › Now place on the pan and cook on both sides until golden.
- › Top with honey or fruit compote.

Feel indulgent with this 'treat' breakfast option to spice up a dull Saturday morning. **Serves 1**

1 egg
25 ml low-fat milk
1 tsp cinnamon
$1/2$ tbsp butter
2 slices of wholemeal bread
$1/2$ tbsp honey or fruit compote

**Calories:**
350

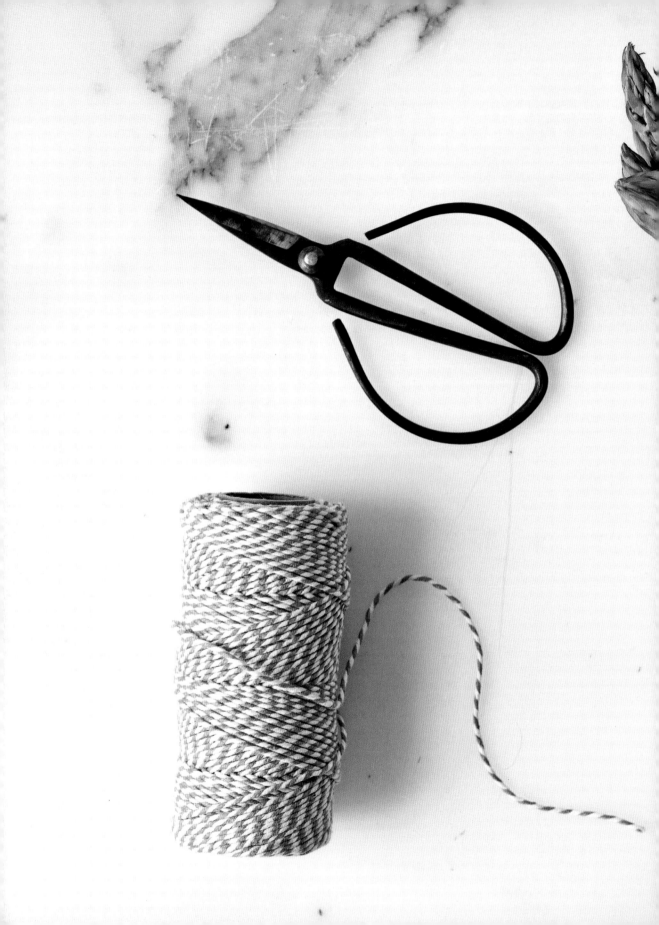

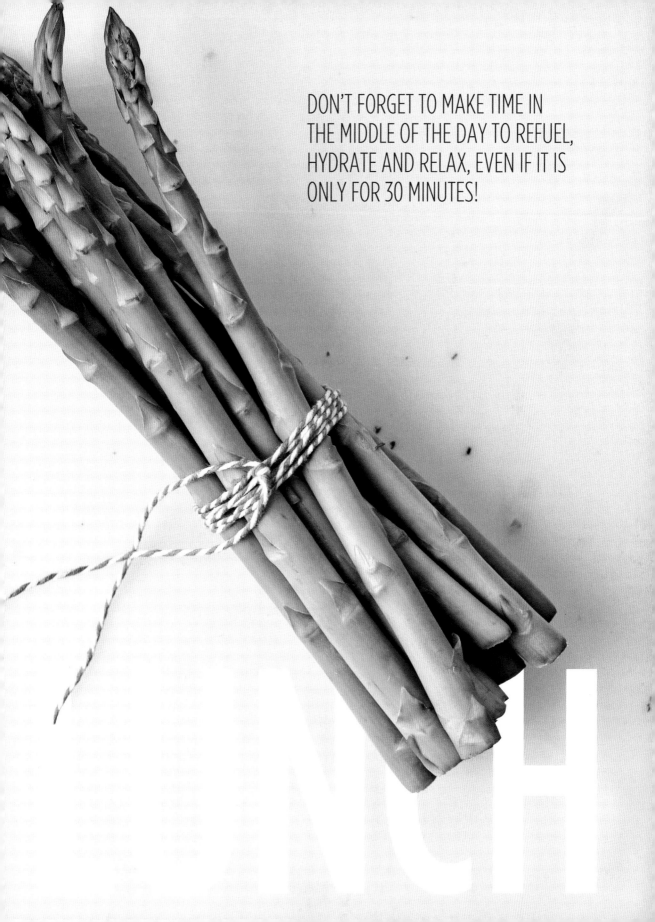

DON'T FORGET TO MAKE TIME IN THE MIDDLE OF THE DAY TO REFUEL, HYDRATE AND RELAX, EVEN IF IT IS ONLY FOR 30 MINUTES!

# SUPER SANDWICHES
## BASE + FILLING

Sandwiches can be super quick and easy at lunch-time. Mix and match the bread options with any of the filling options listed for a tasty lunch-time meal. **Serves 1**

**Bases:**
› 1 wholemeal/wholewheat pitta bread (oval 67 g)
› 1 wholemeal/wholewheat wrap (67 g)
› 2 slices wholemeal/wholewheat bread (74 g)
› 2 slices McCambridge bread (74 g)

**Fillings:**
› Hot Chicken
› Chicken Salad
› Baked Ham and Cheese
› Turkey Club
› Salmon and Dill Mayo

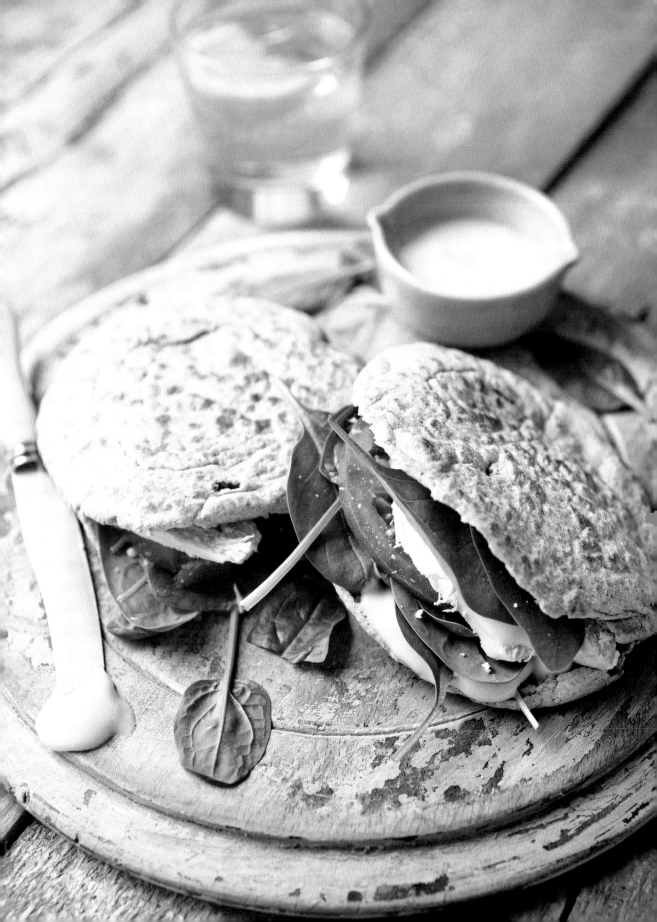

# HOT CHICKEN

base of your choice
1 tbsp salad cream
100 g cooked chicken
   (or leftovers), sliced
1 tomato, sliced
50 g spinach
pinch of pepper

**Calories:**
433

> Spread the base of your choice with salad cream.
> Fill with the cooked chicken, tomatoes and spinach. Top with pepper, if liked.

# CHICKEN SALAD

base of your choice
1 tsp mayonnaise
50 g spinach
1/2 stick of celery, chopped
50 g cherry tomatoes, halved
100 g cooked chicken
   (or leftovers), sliced

**Calories:**
395

> Spread your base of choice with 1 teaspoon of mayonnaise.
> Top with the spinach, celery, tomatoes and cooked chicken.

# BAKED HAM AND CHEESE

› Spread your chosen base with mustard and top with ham, tomato and onion.
› Place under the grill until golden brown.
› Then remove from the grill, sprinkle cheese on top. Return to the grill until the cheese has melted.

base of your choice
½ tsp mustard
75 g cooked ham
1 tomato, sliced
¼ onion, sliced
20 g Cheddar cheese, grated

**Calories:**
386

# TURKEY CLUB

› Place your base of choice on a plate and spread with salad cream.
› Wash and dry the tomato and salad leaves.
› Cut the tomato into slices and place on the bread, followed by the turkey and salad leaves.

base of your choice
1 tbsp salad cream
1 tomato
50 g mixed salad leaves
100 g cooked turkey (or use leftovers)

**Calories:**
437

# SALMON AND DILL MAYO

1 tsp dill, stemmed
2 tsp mayonnaise
base of your choice
60 g smoked salmon
½ cucumber, thinly sliced

**Calories:**
436

› To make the dill mayo, bring a saucepan of water to the boil. Add the dill and stir for 10–15 seconds.
› Drain and transfer to a bowl of ice water to cool.
› Squeeze dry with your hands or paper towels, and purée in a blender.
› Add the mayonnaise to the puréed dill and spread on your base of choice.
› Add the smoked salmon and top with the cucumber.

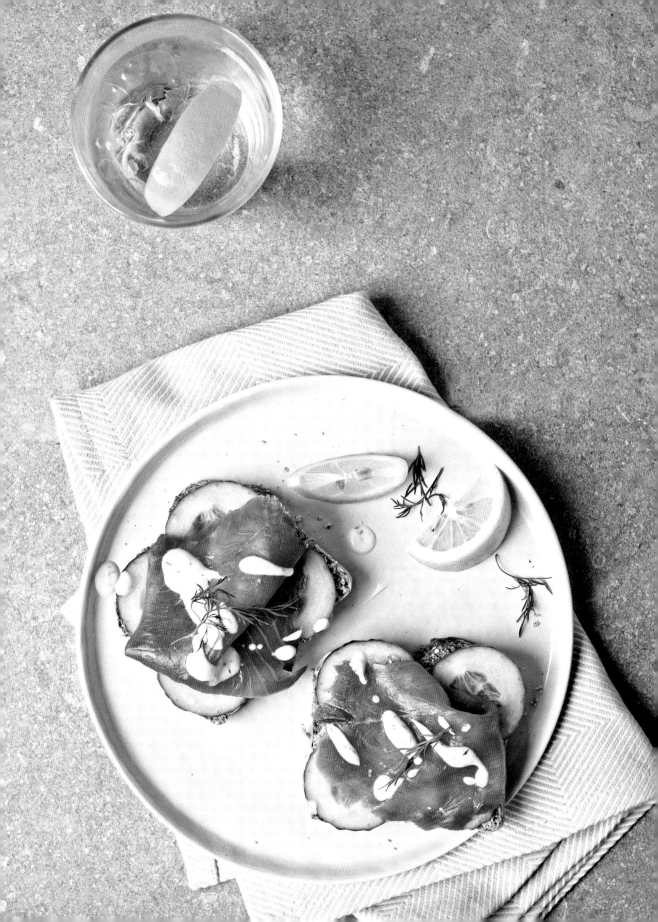

# MID-WEEK LUNCH-TIME STAPLES: SOUP AND SANDWICHES

Some of my 'go to' lunch options combine my favourite foods: soup and sandwiches. Prepare the soup ahead of time and freeze in 200 ml portions to ensure this a quick option at lunch time and the perfect accompaniment to any sandwich.

BASE OPTIONS:
1 slice wholemeal bread
2 Ryvita crackers

FILLING OPTIONS:
turkey club
baked ham and cheese
salmon and dill mayo

SOUP OPTIONS:
sweet potato and celery
minestrone
carrot and coriander

## Calories:
200 ml soup and turkey club 352
200 ml soup and baked ham and
   cheese 386
200 ml soup and salmon and dill
   mayo 304

› Top the base of your choice with the filling of your choice.
› Serve with a cup (200 ml) of sweet potato, minestrone or carrot and coriander soup.

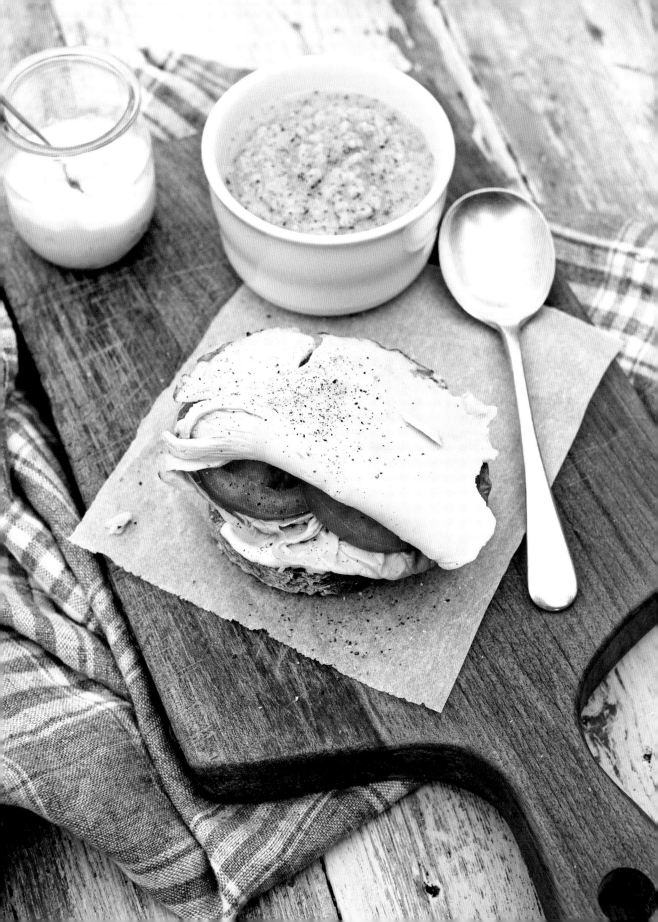

I love, love, love soup. I find it so comforting in winter or summer. Here are a few options for you to get your tastebuds around! A good tip is to make these ahead and freeze in 200 ml and 400 ml portions so that you can have a quick snack or lunch at any time.

# SOULFUL SOUPS
# CHICKEN NOODLE SOUP

This is one of my favourite soups – quick, tasty and oh so easy!

**Serves 3 x 600 ml**

1 tbsp rapeseed oil
2 carrots, chopped
1 onion, finely chopped
2 sticks of celery, sliced
950 ml reduced-sodium chicken stock (use 2 stock cubes)
500 ml water
1 tsp dried thyme
90 g wholewheat fusilli pasta
150 g cooked chicken (or leftovers), cut into chunks

**Calories:**
282

› Heat the oil in a large pot over a medium heat.
› Add the carrots, onion and celery.
› Mix the chicken stock and add a further 500 ml of water. Add this stock mixture to the pot.
› Now add the thyme, pasta and cooked chicken.
› Bring to the boil, reduce the heat to medium and simmer for 10–15 minutes, or until the pasta is cooked.

# SWEET POTATO AND CELERY SOUP

› Put the sweet potato, celery and turnip into a large pot.
› Add the water and bring to the boil. Then turn down the heat and simmer until completely tender, about 30–45 minutes.
› Heat the oil in a separate pan over a medium heat. Add the onion, stirring often until soft.
› Add the softened onion to the pot and stir in the thyme, vegetable stock, nutmeg and allspice. Simmer for 5 minutes.
› Using a hand blender or a food processor, blend the mixture until smooth.

This is a thick soup, so add some water if you prefer it a bit thinner.
**Serves 4 x 400 ml**

450 g sweet potato, peeled and diced
225 g celery, diced
170 g turnip, peeled and diced
600 ml water
1 tbsp olive oil
1 onion, chopped
1 tsp dried thyme
475 ml reduced-sodium vegetable stock
$1/4$ tsp nutmeg
pinch of ground allspice

**Calories:**
186

# BUTTERNUT SQUASH AND VEGETABLE SOUP

Butternut squash is a great base for soup – you can mix and match with other in-season vegetables to change up this recipe over the year.

**Serves 4 x 400 ml**

600 ml reduced-sodium
   vegetable stock
350 g butternut squash, peeled
   and chopped
1 courgette, chopped
1 cauliflower, chopped
1 tbsp tomato purée

**Calories:**
100

› Pour the vegetable stock into a large pot and place over a medium heat.
› Add all the chopped vegetables and the tomato purée.
› Bring to the boil and then turn down to a simmer for 20–25 minutes, until all the vegetables are soft.
› For a smooth soup, use a hand blender or food processor and blend the vegetable mixture.

# CREAM OF BROCCOLI SOUP

› Heat the oil in a large pot over a medium heat.
› Add the leeks, stirring often until tender.
› Add the stock and beans, and bring to a simmer.
› Then add the broccoli and cook until tender, about 5–7 minutes.
› Working in batches, purée the soup using a food processor or a hand blender. (Return the soup to the pot if you have used a food processor.)
› Add the lemon zest and juice, and season with pepper and salt, if liked.
› Place over a medium to high heat until warm enough to serve.
› Garnish with the Parmesan shavings.

Cannellini beans add the 'cream' to this soup. A cheat, but still tasty!
**Serves 3 x 400 ml**

1 tbsp olive oil
50 g leek, white part only, sliced
660 ml reduced-sodium vegetable stock
1 x 400g tin cannellini beans, drained and rinsed (240 g when drained)
400 g broccoli, chopped
$\frac{1}{2}$ tsp lemon zest
1 tbsp lemon juice
pinch of salt and pepper
22 g Parmesan cheese, shaved

**Calories:**
237

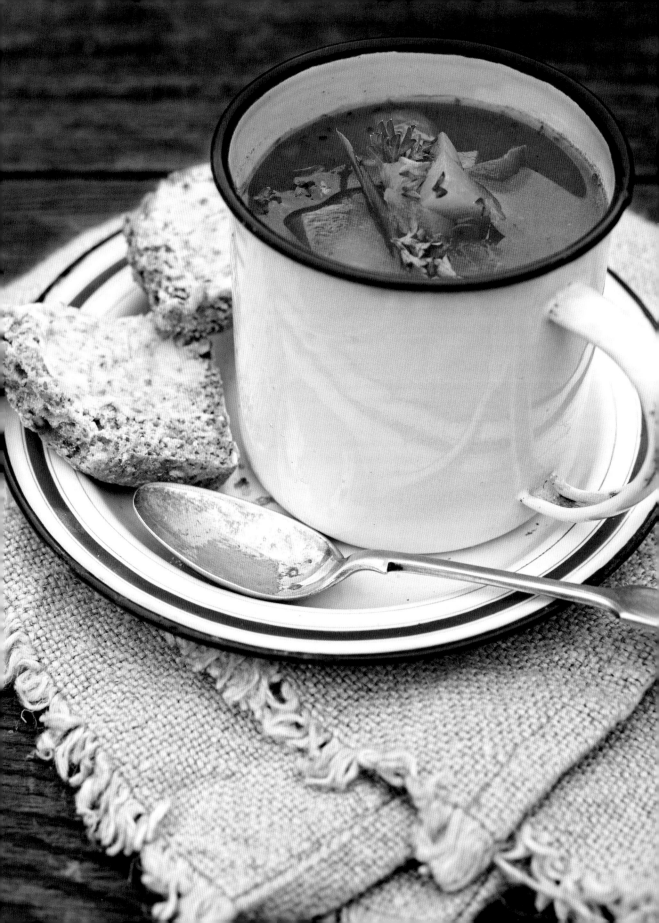

# MINESTRONE SOUP

› Heat the oil in a large pot and add the onion. Sauté for 10 minutes until soft.
› Add the carrots, peppers, chilli pepper, garlic, celery, stock, tomatoes and tomato purée.
› Cook for 15–20 minutes, or until the vegetables are just cooked. Add the chickpeas and cook for a further 5 minutes.
› Add the oregano and thyme, and serve hot.

A traditional favourite – great in winter or summer!
**Serves 5 x 400 ml**

1 tsp olive oil
2 onions, chopped
2 carrots, chopped
1 red pepper, deseeded and chopped
1 yellow pepper, deseeded and chopped
1 red chilli pepper, finely sliced
4 cloves of garlic, finely sliced
2 sticks of celery, chopped
1000 ml reduced-sodium chicken or vegetable stock
1 × 400 g tin chopped tomatoes
1 tsp tomato purée
1 × 400 g tin chickpeas, drained and rinsed (240 g when drained)
2 sprigs oregano
1 tsp dried thyme

**Calories:**
157

# CARROT AND CORIANDER SOUP

This is an easy soup to make at weekends if carrots are part of your Sunday roast. It means you only have to peel carrots once but get double the benefit! **Serves 5 x 400 ml**

4 tsp butter
2 onions, chopped
1 potato, peeled and chopped
6 carrots, chopped
1000 ml reduced-sodium vegetable stock
2 tbsp chopped coriander

**Calories:**
136

› Melt the butter in a large pot on a medium heat. Add the onion and sauté until soft.
› Add the potato and carrots, and toss until well coated.
› Pour in the stock and bring to the boil. Then lower the heat and simmer for 20 minutes, until the vegetables are tender.
› Add the coriander and serve hot.

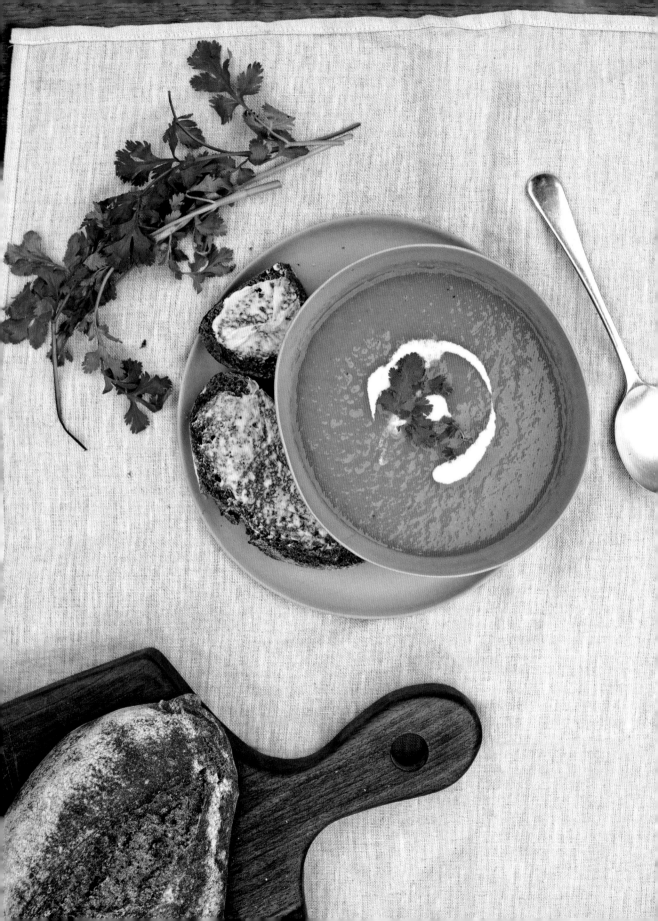

# HEARTY CHICKPEA SOUP

This hearty soup bowl is a meal in itself. **Serves 1 x 600 ml**

1 tbsp olive oil
1 small onion, chopped
1 stick of celery, chopped
1 clove of garlic, crushed
1 tsp cumin
300 ml reduced-sodium
    vegetable stock
200 g tinned chopped tomatoes
115 g tinned chickpeas, drained
    and rinsed
50 g frozen peas
juice and zest of ¹/₂ lemon
freshly ground black pepper
1 tbsp chopped parsley

**Calories:**
416

› Heat the oil in a large pot and then add the onion, celery and garlic.
› Cook on a medium heat for 10 minutes, making sure to stir regularly.
› Add the cumin and cook for a further minute.
› Add the stock, tomatoes and chickpeas, and bring back to the boil. Then simmer for 10 minutes.
› Add the peas and lemon juice. Season with black pepper to taste.
› Top with lemon zest and parsley.

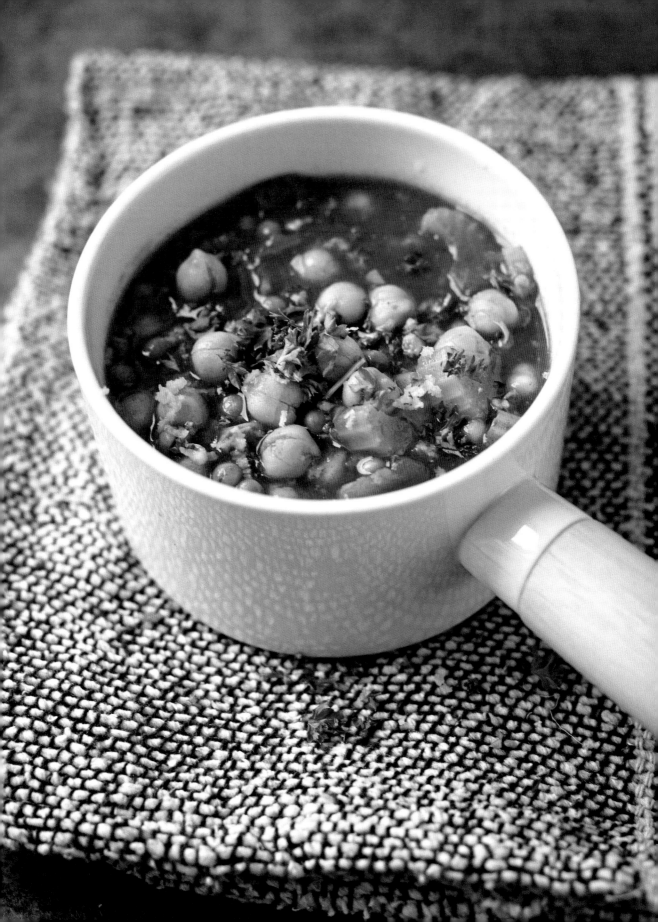

# CHICKEN AND LENTIL SOUP

Another hearty soup that is great for lunch. **Serves 1 x 600 ml**

$^1/_2$ carrot, chopped
$^1/_2$ parsnip, chopped
$^1/_2$ turnip, peeled and chopped
1 stick of celery, chopped
400 ml reduced-sodium
   vegetable stock
100 g chicken breast, cut into
   chunks
40 g red lentils

**Calories:**
351

› Place all the vegetables, stock, chicken and lentils in a large pot and bring to the boil.
› Turn down the heat and simmer until the chicken is cooked through and the vegetables soft.
› You can blend this if you prefer a smooth soup, or leave it chunky.
› Serve hot.

# PEA AND MINT SOUP

› Heat the oil in a large pot and fry the onions and garlic for 2 minutes.
› Add the peas and allow to soften, about 2 minutes.
› Stir in the chopped mint leaves and cook for a minute.
› Then add the vegetable stock and bring to the boil.
› Reduce the heat and simmer uncovered for 15–20 minutes.
› Blend the cooked mixture in a food processor. Season with a little salt and pepper.

This is a great summer soup.

**Serves 2 x 400 ml**

1 tbsp olive oil
2 onions, finely chopped
2 cloves of garlic, finely chopped
500 g frozen peas
bunch of mint, chopped
500 ml reduced-sodium
    vegetable stock
pinch of salt and pepper

**Calories:**
324

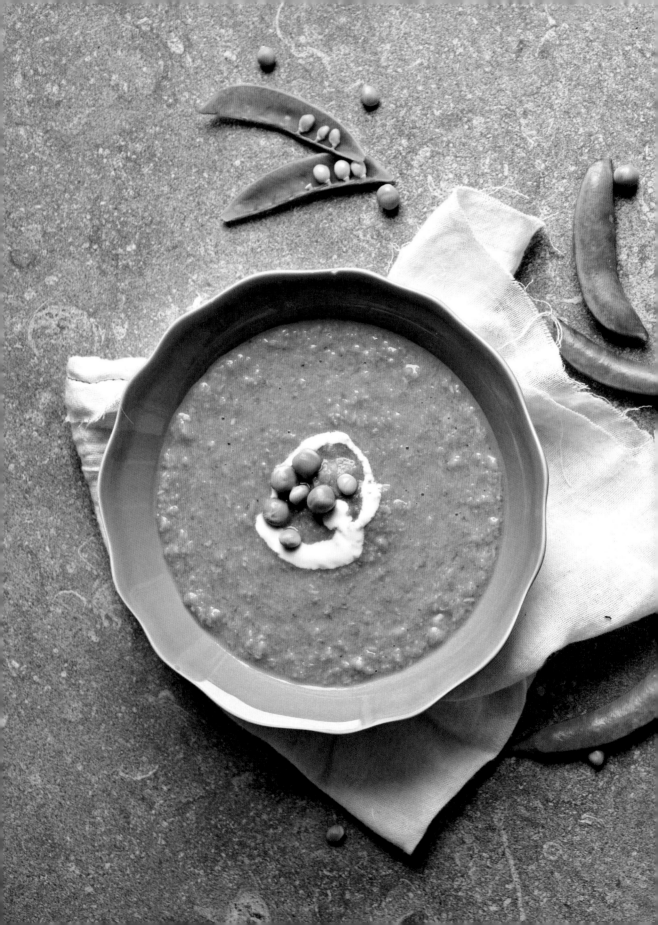

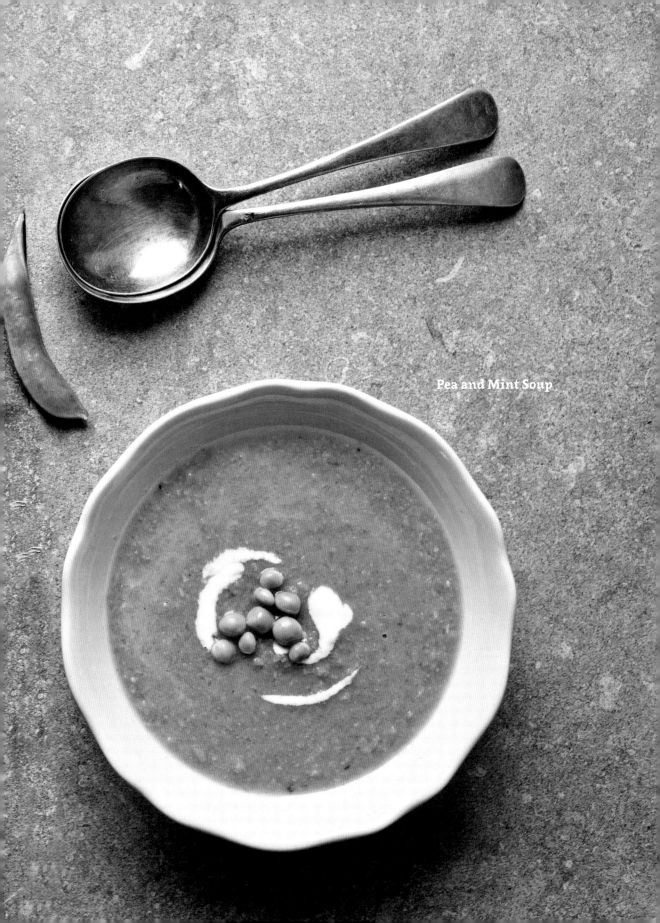

Pea and Mint Soup

Lunch can often be a dull affair. Try some of these salads to spice things up in the middle of the day!

# SASSY SALADS
# TEMPTING TURKEY SALAD AND CRISP BREAD

This recipe is perfect for using leftover turkey from a special occasion. **Serves 1**

2 slices of wholemeal crisp bread
$^1/_2$ tbsp butter (optional)
65 g spinach
$^1/_2$ red pepper, deseeded and chopped
1 tomato, chopped
$^1/_4$ cucumber, thinly sliced
75 g cooked turkey (or use leftovers), thinly sliced
1 tbsp vinaigrette salad dressing (optional) (page 209)

**Calories:**
390

› Lightly butter the crisp bread, if liked.
› In a large bowl layer the spinach, pepper, tomato and cucumber.
› Add the cooked turkey.
› Serve with vinaigrette salad dressing.

# TANTALISING TUNA SALAD

› Bring the water to the boil in a pot. Add the couscous and cover until cooked.
› Place the salad leaves, spinach, pepper, carrot and cherry tomatoes in a large bowl.
› Mix the raisins with the couscous and add to the salad.
› Top with tuna and serve with balsamic vinegar, if liked.

Tuna is a quick option for adding protein to lunch. **Serves 1**

60 ml water
25 g couscous
25 g butterhead lettuce
25 g spinach
$1/2$ red pepper, deseeded and chopped
$1/2$ carrot, grated
50 g cherry tomatoes, halved
10 g raisins
75 g tuna, drained and flaked
1 tbsp balsamic vinegar

**Calories:**
350

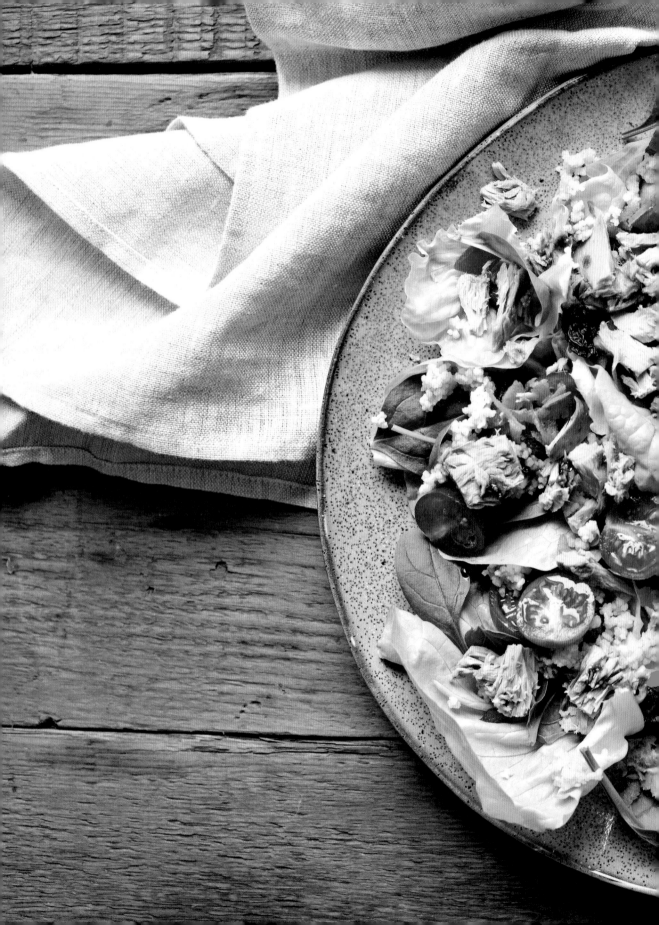

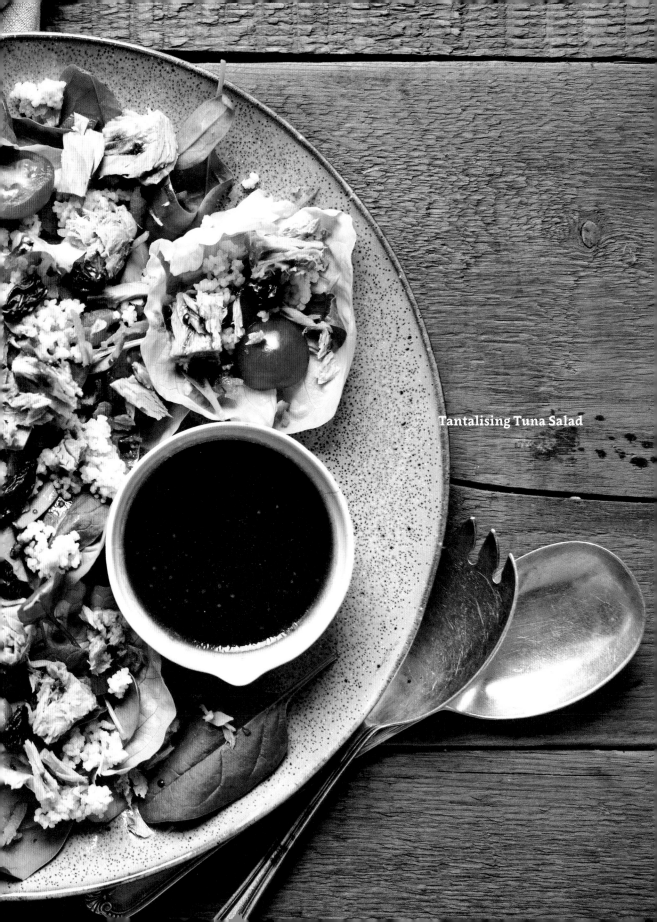

Tantalising Tuna Salad

# BBQ CHICKEN SALAD

One of my favourite salads. This salad can be a nice light option for dinner too. **Serves 1**

50 g salad leaves
50 g spinach
100 g cherry tomatoes, halved
75 g cooked chicken (or leftovers), chopped
25 g black-eyed beans
50 g sweetcorn
$1/4$ cucumber, thinly sliced
1 spring onion, chopped
20 g Cheddar cheese, grated
1 tbsp chopped coriander
2 tbsp BBQ sauce

**Calories:**
380

› Place the salad leaves, spinach and tomatoes on a plate.
› Top with the chopped chicken, black-eyed beans, sweetcorn, cucumber, spring onion, cheese and coriander.
› Drizzle with the BBQ sauce.

# TUNA PANZANELLA SALAD

› Preheat the grill to medium low.
› Brush the bread with 1 teaspoon of oil.
› Grill the bread until lightly toasted, about 2 minutes per side.
› Cut the toasted bread into cubes and transfer to a large bowl.
› Add the tomatoes, cucumber, salad leaves, spinach, basil, capers, balsamic vinegar and remaining oil.
› Top with the tuna and serve.

Panzanella is a bread and tomato salad. Did you know there are over 3,000 varieties of tomato? **Serves 1**

1 slice of crusty wholegrain bread
2 tsp olive oil
2 tomatoes, chopped
$1/2$ cucumber, thinly sliced
50 g salad leaves
50 g spinach
bunch of basil, chopped
$1^1/_2$ tsp capers
$1^1/_2$ tsp balsamic vinegar
56 g tuna, drained and flaked

**Calories:**
338

# SUNSHINE SALAD

A nice vegetarian salad option.

**Serves 1**

50 g salad leaves
50 g yellow split peas
700 ml water
$^1/_4$ tsp cumin
1 tsp lemon juice
1$^1/_2$ tsp olive oil
20 g pineapple, peeled and
   chopped
1 tbsp chopped parsley
1 tbsp chopped mint

**Calories:**
200

› Wash and dry the salad leaves, if necessary, and place on a plate.
› Put the split peas into a saucepan with the 700 ml of water and cumin. Bring to the boil and then simmer, covered, for about 20 minutes, until tender. Keep an eye on them so they don't turn to mush.
› While the split peas are still warm, stir in the lemon juice and oil.
› Stir in the remaining ingredients.
› Top the leaves with the split pea mixture.

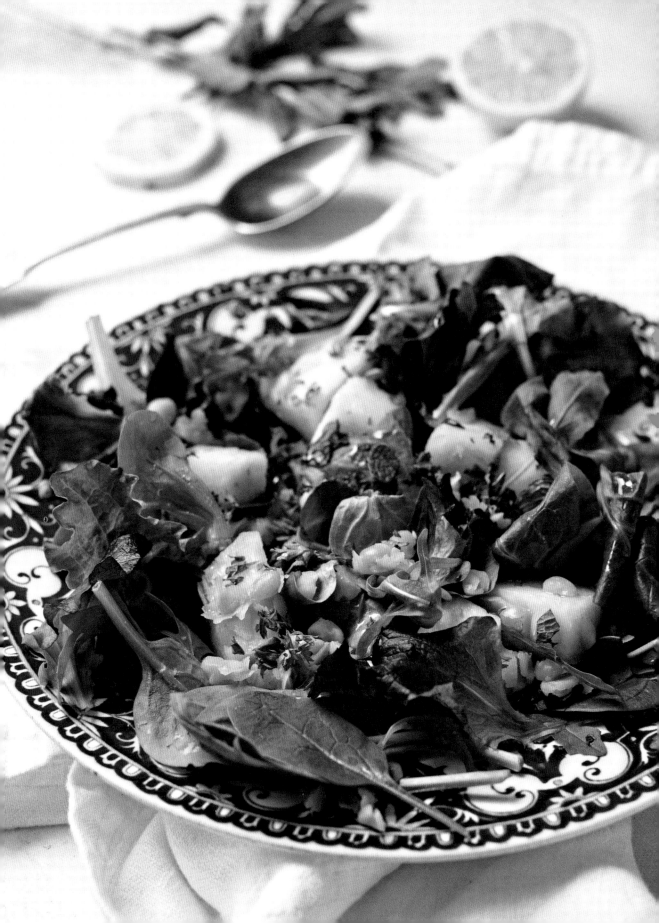

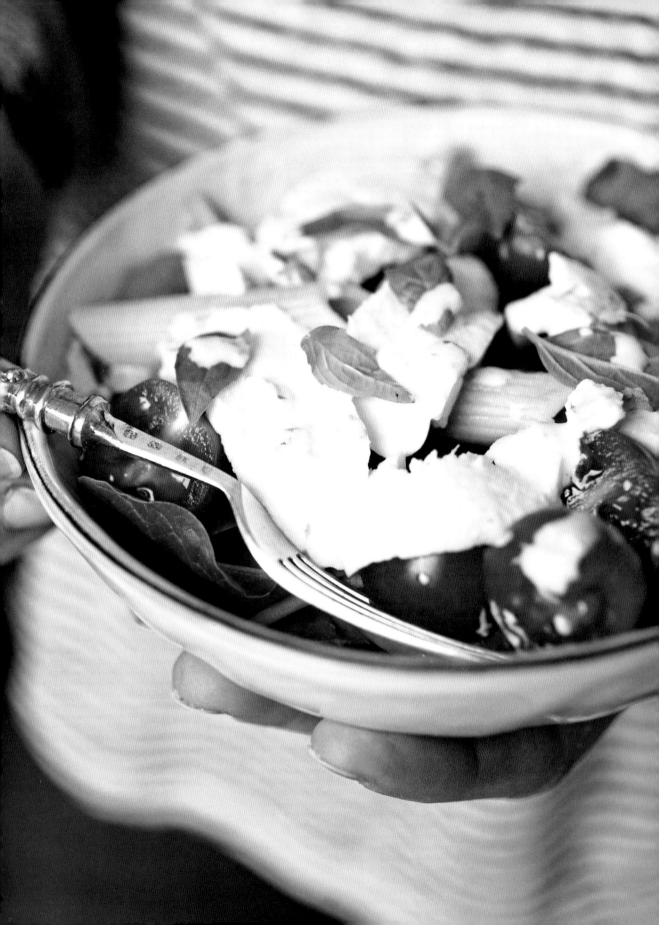

# CAPRESE PASTA SALAD

› Add the pasta to a pot of water. Bring to the boil and simmer until cooked. Drain and rinse in cold water.
› In a small bowl, mix the yogurt, lemon juice and pesto.
› Combine the mozzarella, tomatoes, basil and cooked pasta, then place on top of the spinach.
› Drizzle with vinaigrette salad dressing.

*A lovely fresh salad – perfect when cherry tomatoes are in season in summer months.* **Serves 1**

30 g wholewheat penne pasta
40 g natural yogurt (3% fat)
juice of $1/4$ lemon
$1/2$ tbsp pesto
40 g mozzarella cheese, sliced
90 g cherry tomatoes, halved
bunch of basil, torn
25 g spinach
1 tbsp vinaigrette salad dressing
   (page 209)

**Calories:**
395

# TOMATO AND AVOCADO SALAD

Avocados are a great source of omega-3 fat – good for your heart and for reducing inflammation.

**Serves 1**

100 g salad leaves
60 g cherry tomatoes, halved
40 g olives, quartered
2 tbsp chopped mint
$^1/_4$ avocado, chopped
2 tbsp vinaigrette salad dressing
  (page 209)

**Calories:**
370

› In a bowl, combine the salad leaves, tomatoes, olives, mint and avocado.
› Drizzle with vinaigrette salad dressing.

# SPINACH SALAD WITH CHICKEN, CORN AND FETA

› Add the chicken to a pot of water and bring to the boil. Then reduce the heat and simmer gently until the chicken is cooked through.
› In a bowl, combine the lemon juice and oil.
› Place the spinach leaves on a plate, top with the chopped tomatoes, sweetcorn and cooked chicken. Scatter feta cheese over the salad.
› Drizzle with the combined lemon and oil dressing.

You can serve the chicken warm in this recipe to make it more appetising on cold days.

**Serves 1**

100 g chicken breast, cut into thin strips
$^{1}/_{2}$ tbsp lemon juice
$^{1}/_{2}$ tbsp olive oil
75 g baby spinach
2 tomatoes, chopped
90 g sweetcorn
15 g feta cheese, crumbled

**Calories:**
398

# BAKED TOMATOES WITH GOAT'S CHEESE

Anything that includes goat's cheese is a favourite of mine. Add it to tomatoes and you're on to a winner! **Serves 1**

2 large tomatoes
2 tsp olive oil
30 g goat's cheese, crumbled
30 g breadcrumbs
1 tsp chopped thyme
1 tsp chopped parsley
zest of $1/2$ lemon

FOR THE SIDE SALAD:
25 g spinach
25 g cherry tomatoes, halved
$1/2$ cucumber, thiny sliced

**Calories:**
388

› Preheat the oven to 220°C/425°F/gas 7.
› Slice the top off the tomatoes and scoop out the seeds. Drizzle each tomato with a half teaspoon of olive oil.
› Fill each tomato with 15 g crumbled goat's cheese.
› Combine the breadcrumbs, 1 teaspoon of olive oil, thyme, parsley and lemon zest.
› Bake until golden brown, about 5 minutes.

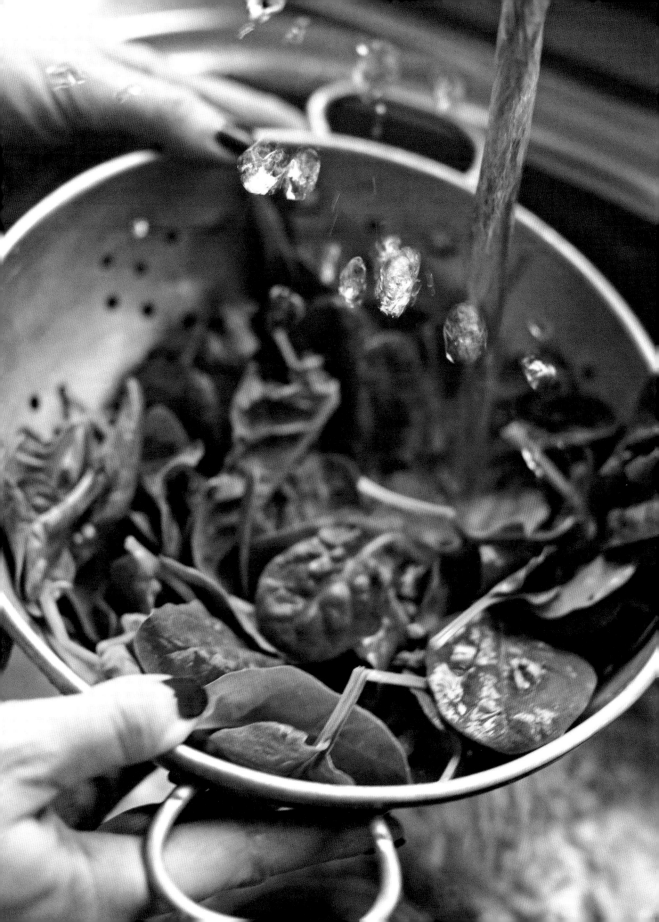

# CAJUN-GRILLED CHICKEN AND BLACK-EYED BEAN SALAD

A Mexican-inspired salad with my favourite herb, coriander!

**Serves 1**

¹/₄ tsp dried oregano
¹/₄ tsp dried thyme
¹/₂ tsp paprika
¹/₄ tbsp cayenne pepper
¹/₂ clove of garlic, crushed
100 g chicken breast
50 g black-eyed beans
1 tomato, chopped
40 g sweetcorn
1 spring onion, chopped
12 g sun-dried tomatoes, chopped
zest and juice of ¹/₂ lime
2 ¹/₂ tbsp chopped coriander
30 g wholegrain rice

**Calories:**
445

› Mix the oregano, thyme, paprika, cayenne pepper and garlic in a bowl and coat the chicken.
› For the bean salad, mix the black-eyed beans, tomato, sweetcorn, spring onion, sun-dried tomatoes, lime zest and juice and coriander in a large bowl.
› Place the rice in a pot of boiling water and cook until light and fluffy.
› Put on the grill at a medium to high heat. Line a grill pan with foil, place the chicken on it and grill for 5–7 minutes on one side. Once golden brown, turn and grill the other side for a further 5–7 minutes, or until completely cooked through.
› Serve the chicken with the rice and the bean salad.

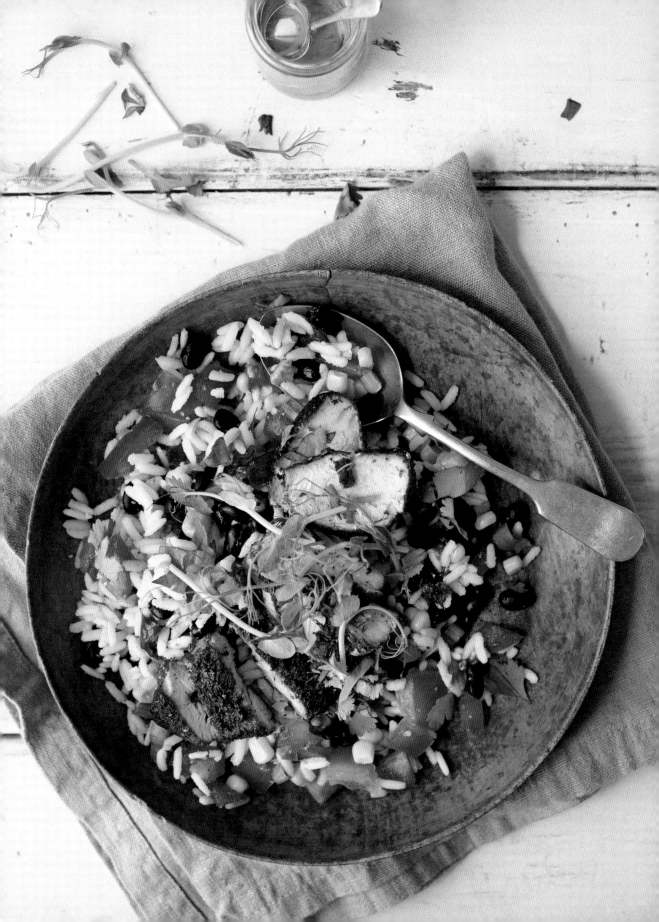

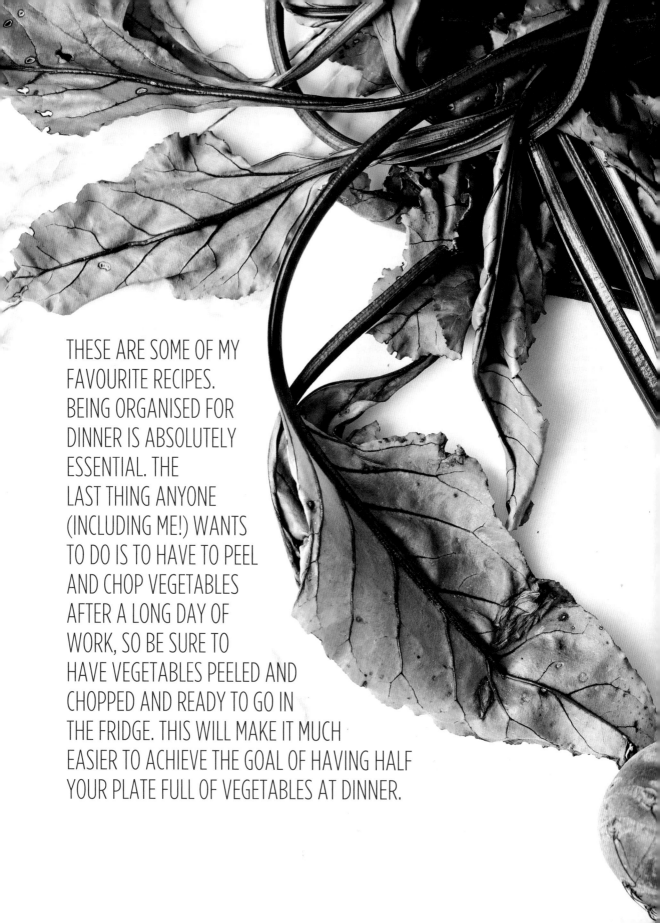

THESE ARE SOME OF MY
FAVOURITE RECIPES.
BEING ORGANISED FOR
DINNER IS ABSOLUTELY
ESSENTIAL. THE
LAST THING ANYONE
(INCLUDING ME!) WANTS
TO DO IS TO HAVE TO PEEL
AND CHOP VEGETABLES
AFTER A LONG DAY OF
WORK, SO BE SURE TO
HAVE VEGETABLES PEELED AND
CHOPPED AND READY TO GO IN
THE FRIDGE. THIS WILL MAKE IT MUCH
EASIER TO ACHIEVE THE GOAL OF HAVING HALF
YOUR PLATE FULL OF VEGETABLES AT DINNER.

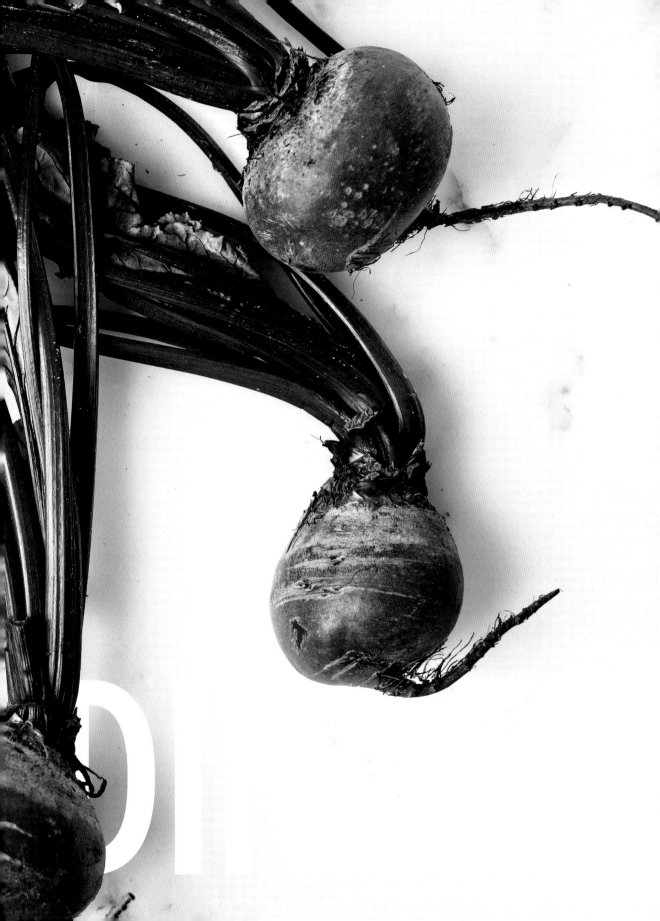

In addition to being a great protein source, red meat is a really important source of iron for the body. You should aim to eat red meat three times a week.

# BEEF
# LASAGNE AND SALAD

A traditional favourite. While this meal takes a bit of effort, the leftovers can be easily frozen in single portions. **Serves 6**

4 tsp olive oil
2 turkey rashers, finely sliced
2 tsp dried or 4 tsp fresh oregano
2 medium onions, finely chopped
2 cloves of garlic, crushed
3 carrots, finely chopped
3 sticks of celery, finely chopped
500 g minced beef
2 x 400 g tin chopped tomatoes
2 tbsp tomato purée
200 ml water
pinch of salt and pepper
bunch of basil, leaves and stalks
    chopped separately
250 g wholewheat lasagne sheets
500 g natural yogurt (3% fat)
50 g Parmesan cheese, grated

FOR THE SIDE SALAD:
150 g salad leaves
3 tomatoes, chopped
1 cucumber, thinly sliced

**Calories:**
554

› Preheat the oven to 190°C/375°F/gas 5. Place 3 teaspoons of oil in a large pan on a medium to high heat.
› Add the turkey rashers and oregano to the pan, and fry until the rashers are lightly cooked.
› Then add the onions, garlic, carrots and celery, and stir.
› Add the minced beef, tinned tomatoes and tomato purée. Add 200 ml of water to the pan.
› Stir in a pinch of salt and pepper and the basil stalks.
› Bring to the boil, then turn down the heat and simmer for 45 minutes, stirring occasionally.
› Add the remaining basil to the sauce.
› Boil some water and pour it into a pan, then add the lasagne sheets with 1 teaspoon of oil for 3–4 minutes to soften.
› Drain the sheets and carefully pat them dry with some kitchen paper to absorb any extra water.
› Spoon ⅓ of the bolognese sauce into the bottom of an ovenproof dish. Layer a sheet of lasagne on top.
› Follow this with ⅓ of the natural yogurt so that it covers the lasagne sheets.
› Repeat this twice more, finishing with a layer of natural yogurt. Top with the grated Parmesan.
› Cover the dish with tinfoil and bake for 20 minutes. After that, remove the foil and cook for a further 30–40 minutes.
› Serve with a side salad of salad leaves, tomatoes and cucumber.

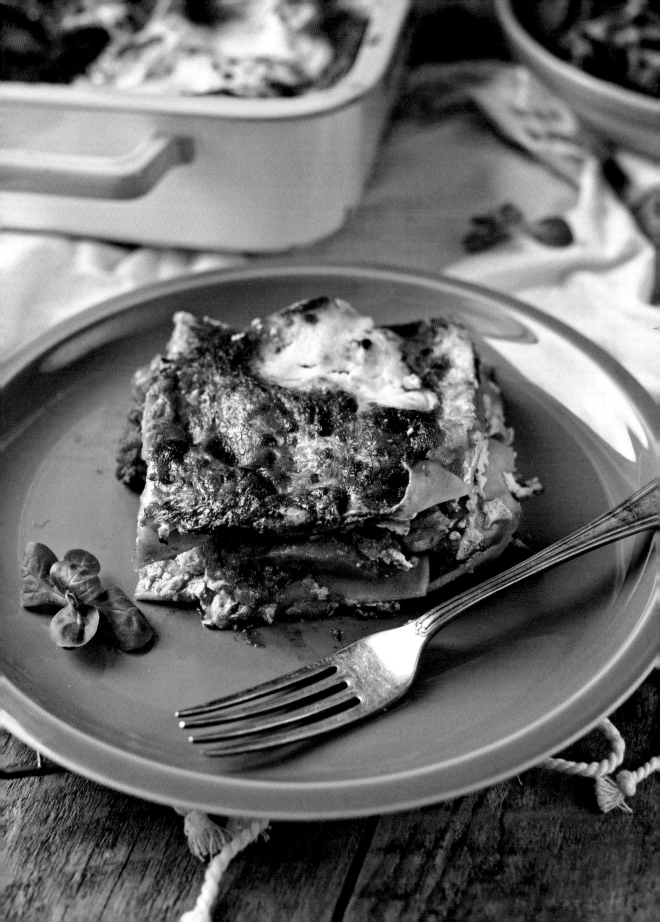

# CURRY BEEF NOODLE BOWL

This is quick and easy. Ask the butcher to cut the steak into strips for you to make this a speedy option for a cold winter evening.

**Serves 2**

200 ml water
100 g wholewheat noodles
1 tbsp rapeseed oil
200 g sirloin steak, cut into strips
1 red pepper, deseeded
   and chopped
1/2 chilli pepper, finely chopped
200 g mushrooms, quartered
2 spring onions, chopped
1 clove of garlic, finely sliced
1 tbsp fish sauce
240 ml reduced-sodium
   chicken stock
2 tbsp curry paste
bunch of basil, chopped, or 3 tsp
   dried basil

**Calories:**
530

› Place 200 ml of cold water in a pot. Add the noodles and bring to the boil. Cover the pot and reduce the heat to a gentle simmer. Cook for 10–20 minutes.
› Over a medium to high heat, add the oil to a pan. Place the beef evenly in the pan.
› Add the pepper, mushrooms and spring onions, and cook for 2–3 minutes until slightly softened.
› Add the garlic, fish sauce, chicken stock and curry paste.
› Simmer for 10–15 minutes. Then add the basil and continue to simmer for a further 1–2 minutes.
› Divide the noodles between two bowls and cover with the beef mixture.

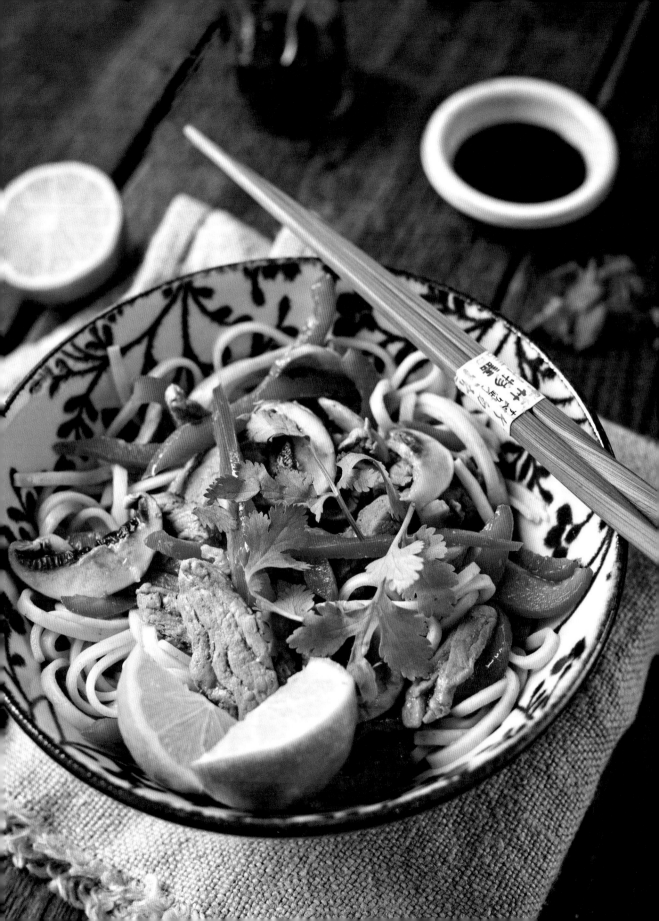

# SPAGHETTI BOLOGNESE

Another traditional favourite and one of my go-to meals. This is an easy meal to prepare ahead of time at the weekend and give yourself a break from cooking on a Monday evening. **Serves 2**

100 g wholewheat spaghetti
2 tbsp olive oil
1 clove of garlic, crushed
1 onion, finely chopped
100 g cherry tomatoes, halved
1 tbsp tomato purée
50 g tinned chopped tomatoes
1/4 tsp salt
2 tsp dried basil
200 g minced beef
1 red pepper, deseeded
  and  chopped
1 green pepper, deseeded
  and chopped
1/2 chilli pepper, finely chopped, or
  1/2 tsp chilli powder

**Calories:**
451

› Place the spaghetti in a pot of cold water and bring to the boil. Turn down the heat and allow to simmer until soft.
› Over a medium heat, add 1 tablespoon of oil to a pot. Add the garlic and onion, and stir until soft.
› Add the chopped cherry tomatoes, tomato purée, tinned tomatoes, salt and basil.
› Simmer on medium heat for 5–10 minutes until the tomatoes are soft, then set aside.
› In a pan, add the the remaining oil and then the minced beef, stirring until brown all over. Drain off the excess juice from the meat.
› Return the pan to the heat and add the peppers and chilli pepper or chilli powder.
› Add the tomato-based sauce and simmer until the peppers are soft.
› Remove the spaghetti from the heat and drain.
› Divide the spaghetti between two plates and ladle on the mince mixture.

# GINGER BEEF

› Put the oil in a pan on a medium to high heat. Add the onion, garlic and pepper, and stir-fry for 5–7 minutes.
› Add the beef and continue to stir-fry for 5 more minutes.
› Add the cumin, lemon juice, ginger and vinegar, and continue to stir as it cooks.
› Then add the broccoli and green beans, and cook until tender.
› While the beef mixture is cooking, put the rice in a pot of boiling water and cook until light and fluffy.
› Divide the rice between two plates and top with the beef mixture.

Ginger is one of my favourite things to add to stir fries as it gives great flavour and also is great for your immune system. **Serves 2**

1 tbsp rapeseed oil
1 onion, sliced
1 clove of garlic, crushed
1 red pepper, deseeded and chopped
250 g sirloin steak, cut into strips
$1/2$ tsp cumin
1 tbsp lemon juice
2 tsp grated ginger
$1 1/2$ tsp white rice vinegar
150 g broccoli florets
150 g green beans
100 g wholegrain rice

**Calories:**
509

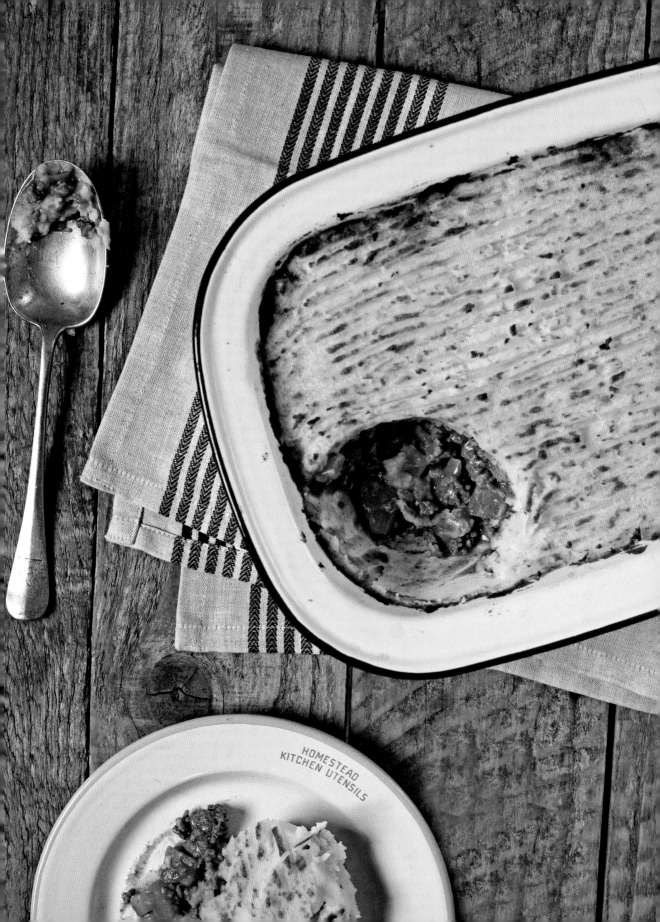

# COTTAGE PIE

› Preheat the oven to 180°C/350°F/gas 4.
› Place the potatoes in a pot with plenty of cold water and bring to the boil. Turn down the heat and simmer until soft.
› Drain the potatoes, add the milk and half of the butter and mash. Set aside for later.
› Melt the remaining butter in a pan and add the onions, celery, carrots and garlic, and cook for 5 minutes until soft.
› Add the minced beef to the pan, stirring until it is brown all over.
› Stir in the flour and cook for 1 minute.
› Add the chicken stock, tomato purée and Worcestershire sauce, and bring to the boil, then turn down the heat and simmer for 5–7 minutes.
› Put the mince mixture into an ovenproof dish and top with the mashed potato.
› Bake for about 30 minutes, until golden on top.

Comfort food all the way! This often tastes better the next day, so leftovers can make a great lunch. If you have it in the house, dissolve 1 tablespoon of Bovril in a little water and add with the stock for a little added flavour. **Serves 4**

500 g potatoes, peeled
50 ml low-fat milk
40 g butter
2 onions, finely chopped
2 sticks of celery, chopped
2 carrots, chopped
2 cloves of garlic, finely chopped
400 g minced beef
25 g flour
500 ml reduced-sodium
   chicken stock
1 tbsp tomato purée
2 tbsp Worcestershire sauce

**Calories:**
517

# BEEF AND RICE

The slower this is cooked, the more tender the meat will be.

**Serves 2**

240 ml reduced-sodium beef stock
240 ml water
2 tsp butter
80 g wholegrain rice
1 tbsp rapeseed oil
225 g sirloin steak, cut into strips
1 large onion, chopped
2 cloves of garlic, crushed
1 green pepper, deseeded
  and chopped
1 red pepper, deseeded
  and chopped
2 tsp Worcestershire sauce
200 g tinned chopped tomatoes
1 tsp cumin
1 tsp five-spice powder
2 tbsp chopped parsley

**Calories:**
545

› Put the beef stock, water and butter in a medium-sized pot, and bring to the boil on a medium to high heat.
› Add the rice, reduce the heat and cover the pot. Cook for 20 minutes, or until the rice is cooked and all the liquid has been absorbed.
› Place a deep skillet/pan on a medium to high heat and add the oil. Add the beef and brown for 2–3 minutes.
› Reduce to a medium heat and add the onion, garlic, peppers and Worcestershire sauce. Cook for a further 7–10 minutes until the vegetables are tender.
› Add the tinned tomatoes, cumin, five-spice and parsley, bring to the boil and then reduce the heat to low and cook for a further 10 minutes.
› Add the cooked rice to the meat and vegetables, and serve hot.

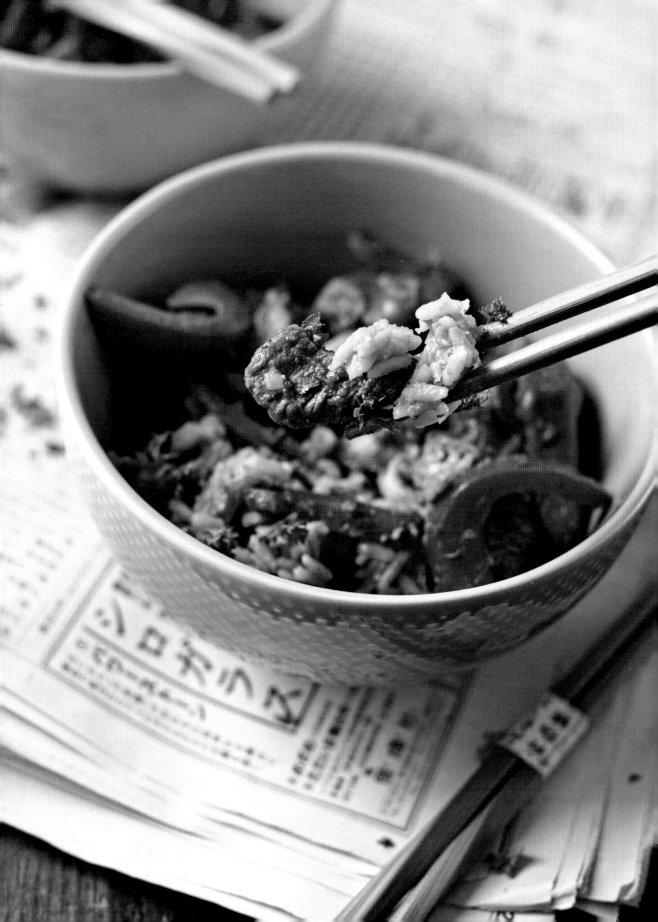

# ITALIAN STEAK

A twist in the sauce means this is lower in fat than many other steak recipes. **Serves 2**

3 tsp rapeseed oil
250 g sirloin steak
pinch of salt and pepper
250 g potatoes
100 g broccoli florets
300 g green beans
150 g tomatoes, chopped
2 cloves of garlic, finely chopped
1 tbsp balsamic vinegar
1 tbsp chopped parsley
1½ tsp dried oregano

**Calories:**
428

› In a frying pan, heat 2 teaspoons of the oil over a medium to high heat.
› Season the steaks with salt and pepper, then place on the pan and cook as desired. (Four minutes per side for medium rare and longer for well done.)
› To a pot of boiling water, add potatoes, and simmer until cooked. Steam the broccoli and green beans.
› In another pot on a medium heat, add 1 teaspoon of oil, along with the tomatoes and garlic, and cook for 5 minutes.
› Then add the balsamic vinegar, parsley and oregano. Cook for a further 3–5 minutes.
› Place each steak on a plate, cover with the tomato mixture, and serve with the potatoes and vegetables.

# MEATBALLS AND SPAGHETTI

› Combine the beef, egg, water, breadcrumbs and onion.
› Roll the mixture into six separate golf ball-sized balls and set aside.
› Heat 1 teaspoon of oil in a pan over a medium to high heat. Once the pan is hot, add the meatballs and cook for 1–2 minutes until browned. Turn the heat down to medium and cook until cooked through.
› Place the spaghetti in a large pot full of boiling water. Turn down the heat and allow to simmer for 10–15 minutes, or until the pasta is tender.
› Put a large pot on a medium heat and add the 1 tablespoon of oil. Add the crushed garlic, stirring gently.
› Quickly add the tomatoes, tomato purée, tinned tomatoes, salt and basil, and mix together.
› Add the chopped peppers, including the chilli powder if using.
› Simmer over a medium heat for 5–10 minutes, until the peppers and tomatoes are soft, and then combine with the cooked meatballs.

A nice change from spag bol! You can prepare these meatballs ahead of time to reduce cooking time.

**Serves 2**

250 g extra lean minced beef
$1/2$ egg
$1/2$ tbsp water
10 g breadcrumbs
1 tbsp onion, finely chopped
1 tsp olive oil
100 g wholewheat spaghetti

FOR THE SAUCE:
3 tsp olive oil
1 clove of garlic, crushed
100 g tomatoes, chopped
1 tbsp tomato purée
50 g tinned chopped tomatoes
$1/4$ tsp salt
2 tsp dried basil
1 red pepper, deseeded and chopped
1 green pepper, deseeded and chopped
$1/2$ chilli pepper, finely chopped, or $1/2$ tsp chilli powder

**Calories:**
552

# POT ROAST

A great option for the slow cooker.
**Serves 4**

3 tsp rapeseed oil
600 g joint of beef
pinch of salt and pepper
1 onion, chopped
6 carrots, chopped
1 small turnip, peeled and chopped
1 clove of garlic, crushed
1 1/2 tsp smoked paprika
1/2 tsp dried thyme
200 g tinned chopped tomatoes
120 ml reduced-sodium beef stock
1 tbsp balsamic vinegar
pinch of saffron
500 g potatoes, peeled
    and quartered

**Calories:**
424

› Preheat the oven to 140°C/275°F/gas 1.
› Heat 1 1/2 teaspoons of oil in a large ovenproof pot, or casserole dish, over a medium to high heat.
› Season the meat with salt and pepper and place into the ovenproof pot or dish. Sear each side until it is nicely browned – this may take about 4 minutes per side.
› Remove the meat and place on a plate.
› Add the remaining oil to the pot and reduce the heat to medium. Add the onion, carrots, turnip, garlic, smoked paprika and thyme, and cook until the vegetables are tender.
› Now add the tomatoes, stock, vinegar and saffron.
› Return the meat to the pot. The vegetables should come about halfway up the sides of the meat.
› Cover the dish, place in the oven and roast for 2 hours.
› Add the potatoes and return to the oven for a further 45–60 minutes, until the meat is cooked through and the potatoes tender.
› Slice the meat and serve with potatoes, vegetables and sauce.

# CHILLI

> Preheat the oven to 190°C/375°/gas 5 and brush a baking tray with 1 teaspoon of olive oil.
> In a bowl, toss the potato and pepper with 2 teaspoons of the oil.
> Season with salt and pepper, if liked, and spread out in a single layer on the baking tray. Roast until tender, about 20–30 minutes.
> In a large pot over a medium to high heat, add 3 teaspoons of oil. Add the onion, stirring often until soft.
> Now stir in the garlic and spices, and cook for a further few minutes.
> Add the minced beef, and cook until it browns. Drain some of the juice from the meat.
> Add the beans, tomatoes, stock and cocoa, and bring to a gentle simmer.
> Add the roasted vegetables and potatoes.
> Serve with a spoonful each of natural yogurt and cheese, and sprinkle with coriander.

A hearty meal for all the family on a cold winter night. **Serves 4**

6 tsp olive oil
1 medium sweet potato, peeled and chopped
1 red pepper, deseeded and chopped
pinch of salt and pepper
$1/2$ onion, chopped
2 cloves of garlic, finely chopped
2 tsp smoked paprika
$1/2$ tsp chilli powder
500 g extra lean minced beef
1 × 400 g tin black beans, rinsed and drained (240 g when drained)
1 × 400 g tin chopped tomatoes
240 ml reduced-sodium chicken stock
1 tbsp unsweetened cocoa powder
40 g natural yogurt (3% fat)
40 g Cheddar cheese, grated
$1/2$ bunch of coriander, chopped

**Calories:**
471

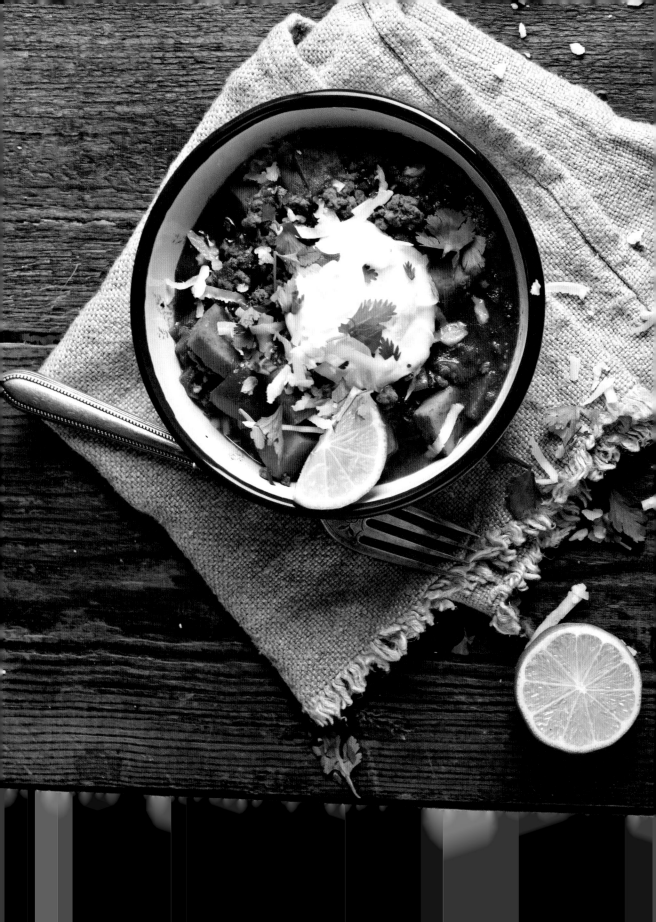

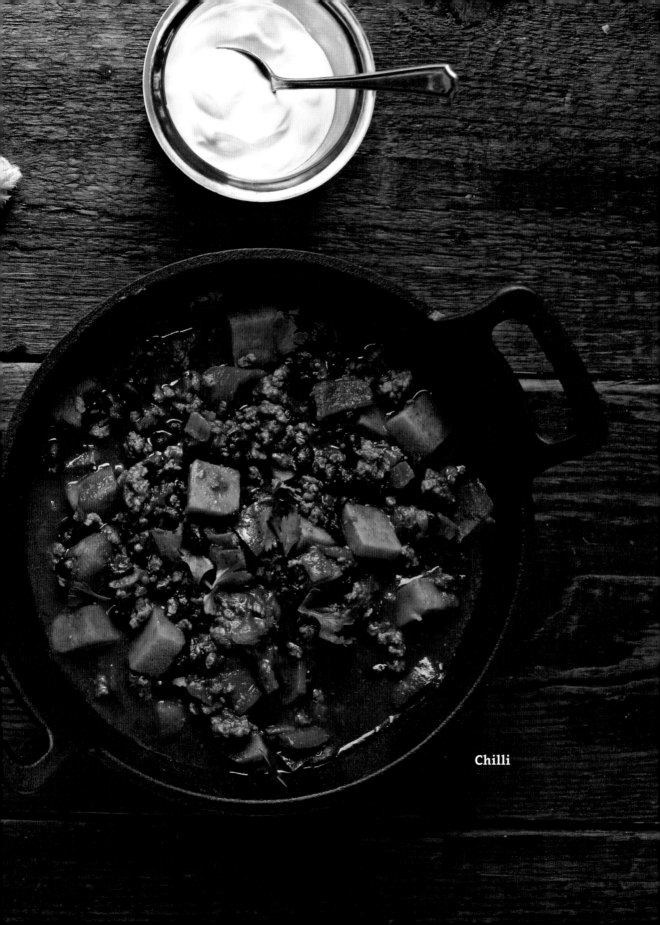

Chilli

# BEEF LO MEIN

You can buy wholewheat noodles in 50 g nests – one less thing to weigh! **Serves 2**

100 g wholewheat noodles
80 ml reduced-sodium
   vegetable stock
1 1/2 tsp reduced-sodium soy sauce
1 tsp cornflour
pinch of pepper
2 tsp rapeseed oil
200 g sirloin steak, cut into
   2.5 cm strips
1/2 tsp garlic, crushed
2 sticks of celery, sliced
2 carrots, sliced
100 g green beans, sliced
100 g bean sprouts
1 x 225 g tin bamboo shoots

**Calories:**
502

› Place the noodles in a pot of water. Bring to the boil, then reduce heat and simmer until cooked.
› In a bowl, combine the stock, soy sauce, cornflour and pepper.
› Heat 1 teaspoon of oil in a pan, or wok, over a medium to high heat. Add the beef and stir until partially cooked, then set aside on a plate.
› Add the other teaspoon of oil to the pan and add all the vegetables. Stir regularly and cook until the vegetables are cooked through but still crisp.
› Add the sauce and meat, and continue to cook until the meat is cooked through.
› Serve with the noodles.

# BUFFALO STEAK AND CORN

› Preheat the oven to 220°C/425°/gas 7.
› Pierce the potatoes 5 or 6 times with a fork and cover with tinfoil. Place on a tray and bake in the oven for 60 minutes, or until cooked through.
› Combine the butter, hot sauce and salt.
› Rub the steak strips with the oil and season with salt and pepper.
› Place in a pan on a medium heat and cook as desired.
› Add the corn to a pot of boiling water and simmer for 5–7 minutes until crisp.
› Remove the baked potatoes from the oven and allow to cool enough to handle.
› Drizzle the hot sauce mixture over the steak and corn, and serve with the potatoes.

Did you know that an average baked potato with skin has more fibre than two slices of wholemeal bread? **Serves 2**

1 $^1/_2$ tbsp butter
1 $^1/_2$ tsp hot sauce
$^1/_4$ tsp salt
250 g sirloin steak, cut into 7.5 cm strips
2 tsp rapeseed oil
pinch of salt and pepper
2 ears of corn
2 medium potatoes

**Calories:**
467

Fish is a great low-saturated fat protein source. It can be a great first protein source for children when solid foods are being introduced (from six months) as the texture is easy to manage. Fish is also a great source of omega-3 fat, which is good for both your heart and your brain!

# FISH
# SEA BASS WITH SALSA-INSPIRED SAUCE

A great tomato-based sauce option for this fish. **Serves 2**

200 ml cold water
100 g wholegrain rice
2 tbsp rapeseed oil
1 red pepper, deseeded
   and chopped
1 green pepper, deseeded
   and chopped
1 onion, chopped
110 g salsa
20 g light cream cheese
2 x 150 g sea bass fillets
pinch of salt and pepper
sprig of parsley (optional)

**Calories:**
557

› Place the 200 ml of cold water in a pot. Add the rice and bring to the boil. Then cover the pot, reduce the heat and simmer for 10–20 minutes until light and fluffy.
› Heat 1 tablespoon of oil in a large pot over a medium heat and add the chopped vegetables. Sauté for 7–10 minutes until tender.
› Add the salsa and light cream cheese to the vegetables, reduce the heat and simmer for a further 5 minutes.
› Season the fish on both sides with salt and pepper.
› Add the remaining oil to a large skillet. Place on a medium to high heat and add the fish.
› Fry the fish on a high heat for 3–4 minutes. Turn over and cook for a further 3–4 minutes on the other side.
› To serve, divide the rice between two plates, layer with the fish and ladle the sauce on top. Garnish with a sprig of parsley, if liked.

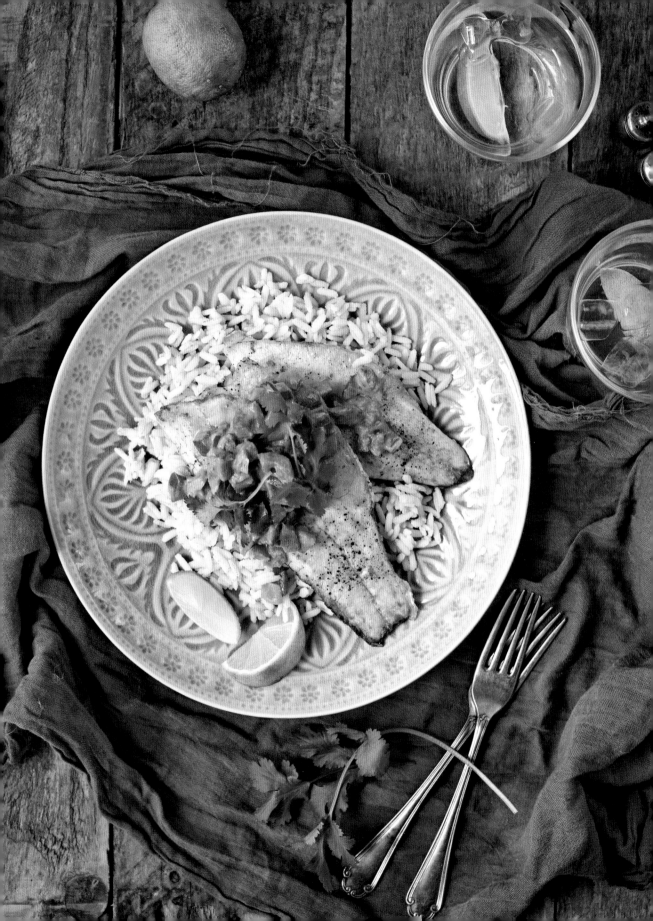

# MEXICAN COD

Quinoa is a nice change from other carbohydrates, but be aware that it does take a little time to prepare.

**Serves 2**

100 g quinoa
300 ml reduced-sodium vegetable
   stock, cold
2 tbsp rapeseed oil
1 red pepper, deseeded
   and chopped
1 yellow pepper, deseeded
   and chopped
1 courgette, chopped
2 tbsp taco spice mix (page 210)
1 tbsp flour
2 x 150 g cod fillets (or any other
   white fish)
2 tbsp chopped coriander
natural yogurt (3% fat)

**Calories:**
526

> Place the quinoa in a pot with the vegetable stock and bring to the boil. Then turn down the heat and simmer for 20 minutes, or until light and fluffy.
> Put 1 tablespoon of the oil in a skillet, or wok, and stir-fry the vegetables on a medium heat until tender.
> Mix the vegetables with the quinoa and set aside.
> Combine the taco spice and flour, and coat the fish with this mixture.
> Heat a pan and add the remaining 1 tablespoon of oil. On a high heat, cook the fish on one side for 4–5 minutes, then turn and cook the other side for 4–5 minutes.
> Divide the quinoa and vegetable mixture between two plates. Place the fish on top and serve.
> Garnish with coriander and natural yogurt, if available.

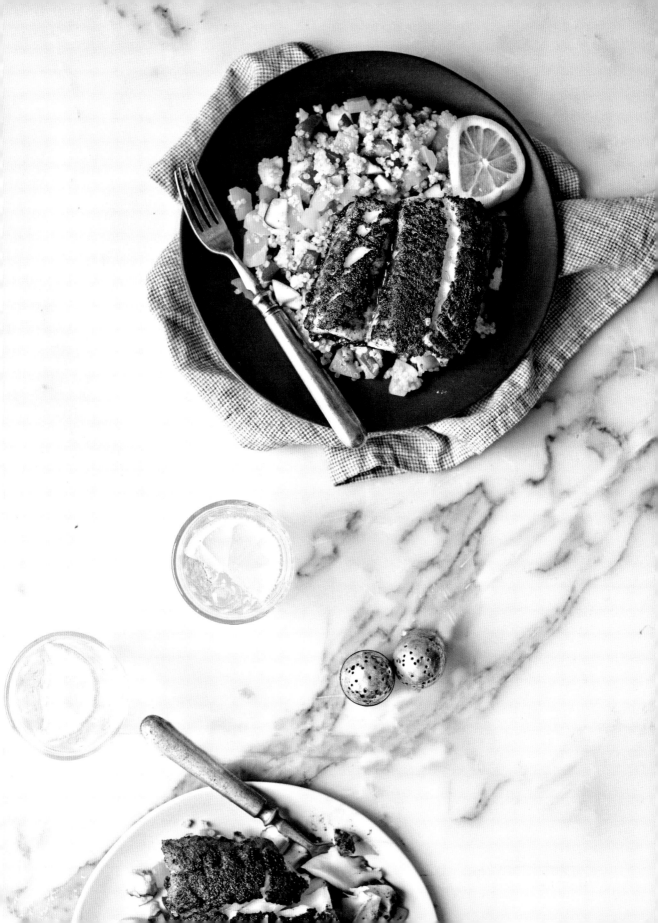

# SUN-DRIED TOMATO SALMON

This can be a super-quick recipe if you keep some salmon in the freezer so that you always have a tasty meal, just minutes away.

**Serves 2**

2 x 120 g salmon fillets
1 tsp sun-dried tomato pesto
   (½ tsp per fillet)
4 sun-dried tomatoes (2 per fillet)
60 g couscous
120 ml reduced-sodium
   vegetable stock, cold
400 g broccoli florets

**Calories:**
540

› Preheat the oven to 200°C/400°F/gas 6.
› Tear off a large piece of tinfoil. Place the salmon fillets on the foil and spread ½ teaspoon of pesto on top of each fillet and top with the sun-dried tomatoes.
› Fold the foil over the fillets, place on a baking tray and put in the oven for 20 minutes, or until cooked through.
› Place the couscous in a pot with the vegetable stock. Bring to the boil, then turn down the heat and simmer for 20 minutes, or until light and fluffy.
› Steam the broccoli florets.
› Remove the fillets from the oven and place on plates. Spoon couscous and broccoli onto each plate and serve.

# SALMON AND COUSCOUS

› Preheat the oven to 200°C/400°F/gas 6.
› Tear off a large piece of tinfoil. Place the salmon fillets in the foil and sprinkle each fillet with 1 teaspoon of paprika.
› Fold the foil over the fillets, place on a baking tray and put in the oven for 20 minutes, or until cooked through.
› Put the couscous in a pot with the vegetable stock. Bring to the boil, then turn down the heat and simmer for 20 minutes, or until light and fluffy.
› Place the oil in a skillet, or wok, on a medium to high heat.
› Add the peppers and courgette, and stir-fry until tender.
› Place the couscous on two plates, cover with the vegetables and top with a salmon fillet each.

A super-quick dish, making it another great mid-week fish option.
**Serves 2**

2 x 120 g salmon fillets
2 tsp paprika
60 g couscous
120 ml reduced-sodium vegetable stock, cold
1 tbsp rapeseed oil
1 red pepper, deseeded and chopped
1 yellow pepper, deseeded and chopped
1 courgette, chopped

**Calories:**
512

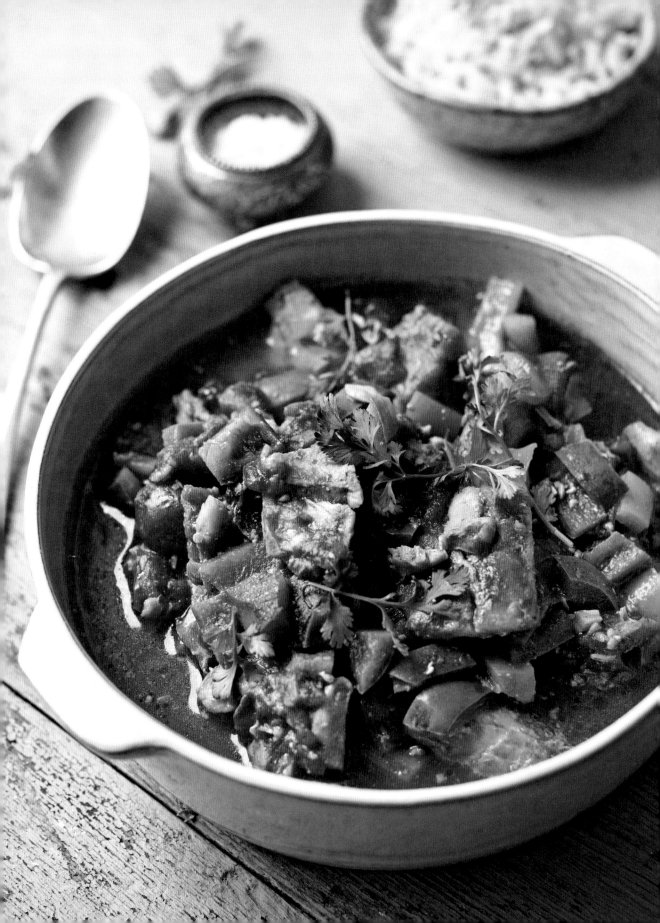

# QUICK FISH STEW

› Fill a pot with 200 ml of cold water, add the rice and bring to the boil. Cover the pot, reduce the heat and gently cook for 10–20 minutes, or until light and fluffy.
› Heat the oil in a pot over a medium heat, then add the garlic and onion, and stir until soft.
› Add the cherry tomatoes, tomato purée, tinned tomatoes, salt and basil. Simmer on medium heat for 5–10 minutes until the tomatoes are soft.
› Add the fish to the tomato sauce, followed by the chopped vegetables.
› Simmer until the fish is cooked and the vegetables tender.
› Divide the cooked rice between two plates and cover with fish stew.

Buying pre-cut fish mix at the fish counter really helps to make this a quick and easy mid-week fish meal.

**Serves 2**

100 g wholegrain rice
1 tbsp olive oil
1 clove of garlic, crushed
$1/2$ onion, finely chopped
100 g cherry tomatoes, halved
1 tbsp tomato purée
100 g tinned chopped tomatoes
$1/4$ tsp salt
1 tsp dried basil
400 g fish pie mix, diced (salmon, white fish, smoked white fish)
1 green pepper, deseeded and chopped
1 yellow pepper, deseeded and chopped

**Calories:**
533

# QUICK TUNA PASTA

A real comfort food for me! Leftovers from this meal can make an ideal lunch the next day.

**Serves 2**

100 g wholewheat penne pasta
25 g butter
25 g flour
200 ml low-fat milk
2 tbsp tomato purée
130 g tuna, drained and flaked
100 g sweetcorn
1 green pepper, deseeded and
    chopped

**Calories:**
496

› Put the pasta in a pot of water, bring to the boil and simmer over a medium heat for 15–20 minutes until tender.
› Melt the butter in a separate pot over a medium heat and stir in the flour.
› Cook for 1 minute and gradually add the milk, stirring continuously to stir to prevent lumps.
› Add the tomato purée and stir for a further minute. Then add the drained tuna, sweetcorn and pepper.
› Finally add the drained, cooked pasta.
› Divide between two plates to serve.

# SEAFOOD CURRY

› Mix the ginger, garlic, cumin and curry paste in a bowl. Stir in the natural yogurt.
› Combine the fish with the spice and yogurt mixture.
› Place the rice in a pot of boiling water and cook until light and fluffy.
› Heat the oil in a large pot and gently fry the onion, cinnamon and bay leaf until the onion is soft.
› Add the fish stock and potatoes, and bring to the boil. Cook for about 20 minutes over a medium heat until the potatoes are tender and the sauce is slightly thicker.
› Now add the fish and yogurt mixture, then reduce the heat to low and cook for 10 minutes until the fish is cooked through.
› Serve with the rice and garnish with the coriander.

Ask the fishmonger to cut the fish into chunks for you and this will save you time when preparing this dish. **Serves 2**

2 tbsp grated or easy ginger
1 clove of garlic, finely chopped
$\frac{1}{2}$ tsp cumin
1 tsp curry paste
75 g natural yogurt (3% fat)
300 g white fish (cod, haddock, monkfish), cut into large chunks
100 g wholegrain rice
1 tbsp rapeseed oil
1 large onion, chopped
$\frac{1}{2}$ tsp cinnamon
1 bay leaf
150 ml reduced-sodium fish stock
250 g potatoes, peeled and chopped
2 tbsp chopped coriander

**Calories:**
557

# MACKEREL AND QUINOA

Mackerel is a great source of omega-3 fatty acids. Mackerel is best eaten when it is in season, during the summer months in Ireland. **Serves 2**

100 g quinoa
300 ml reduced-sodium vegetable stock, cold
1 carrot, grated
1 beetroot, grated
2 × 150 g mackerel fillets

**Calories:**
530

› Preheat the oven to 200°C/400°F/gas 6.
› Put the quinoa in a pot with the vegetable stock. Bring to the boil, then turn down the heat and simmer for 20 minutes, or until light and fluffy.
› Add the grated carrot and beetroot.
› Wrap the mackerel fillets in tinfoil and place in the oven for 15 minutes.
› Place the quinoa and vegetable mixture on two plates and top with mackerel.

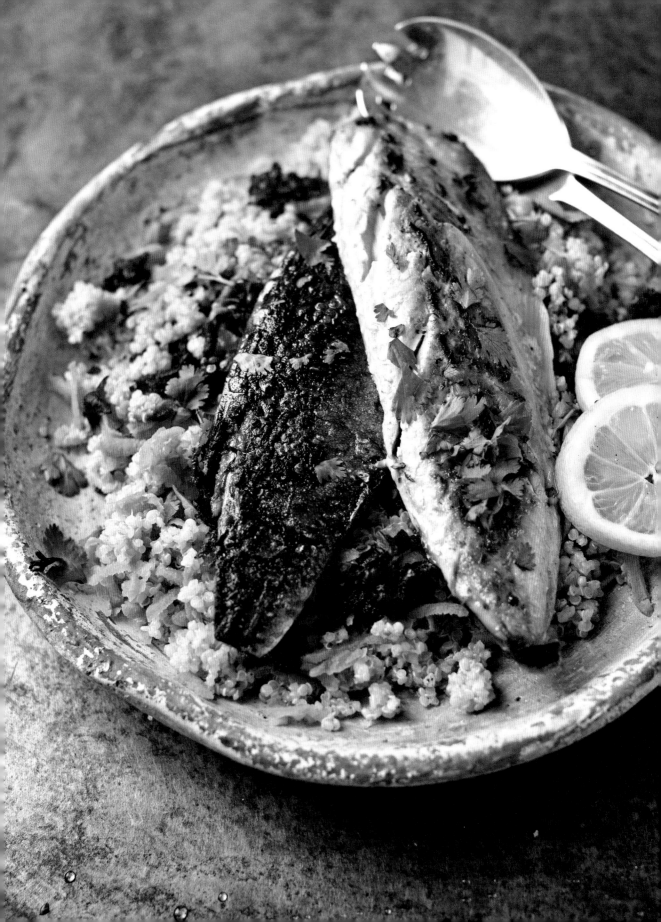

# HADDOCK WITH COCONUT RICE

This can be a great option for the BBQ in summer. **Serves 2**

2 stalks of lemongrass
300 g haddock, cut into cubes
bunch of spring onions, chopped
1 1/2 tbsp rapeseed oil
1/2 tsp chilli flakes
1 clove of garlic, finely chopped
100 g wholegrain rice
100 ml coconut milk
100 ml low-fat milk
100 ml boiled water, slightly cooled
1 tbsp rice wine vinegar
100 g baby spinach

**Calories:**
426

› Slice each of the lemongrass stalks in half lengthwise. Cut the thin ends of each stalk to a point and thread the fish pieces onto these skewers.
› Separate the green and white parts of the spring onions.
› Heat the oil in a large pan with the chilli flakes, garlic and white part of the spring onion.
› Add the fish skewers to the pan and fry gently for about 5 minutes, turning until cooked through.
› Add the rice, coconut milk and low-fat milk to the pan, and bring to the boil.
› Reduce the heat, cover with a lid and cook gently for 8–10 minutes, stirring frequently, until the rice is almost tender and the milk absorbed.
› Add the water, cover and cook for a further 10 minutes, or until the rice is completely cooked.
› Stir in the vinegar, remaining spring onion and spinach.
› Place the cooked rice on two plates and top each one with a fish skewer.

# TERIYAKI SALMON AND CORIANDER RICE

› Preheat the oven to 200°C/400°F/gas 6.
› Put the soy sauce, ginger and chilli sauce in a dish and mix together. Lay the salmon fillets in the marinade and set aside while you prepare the vegetables.
› Put the rice in a pot of boiling water and cook until light and fluffy.
› Steam the asparagus and broccoli.
› Lay the salmon, topped with the marinade and sesame seeds, in a tinfoil parcel and place on a baking tray in the oven. Cook for 15–20 minutes until the fish is cooked through.
› Stir the chopped spring onions and coriander through the rice, and serve with the salmon.

Marinate the salmon fillets overnight to add more flavour to this meal.
**Serves 2**

2 tbsp reduced-sodium soy sauce
2 tsp grated ginger
2 tbsp sweet chilli sauce
2 × 120 g salmon fillets
150 g asparagus
250 g broccoli florets
100 g wholegrain rice
1 tsp sesame seeds
2 spring onions, chopped
2 tbsp chopped coriander

**Calories:**
549

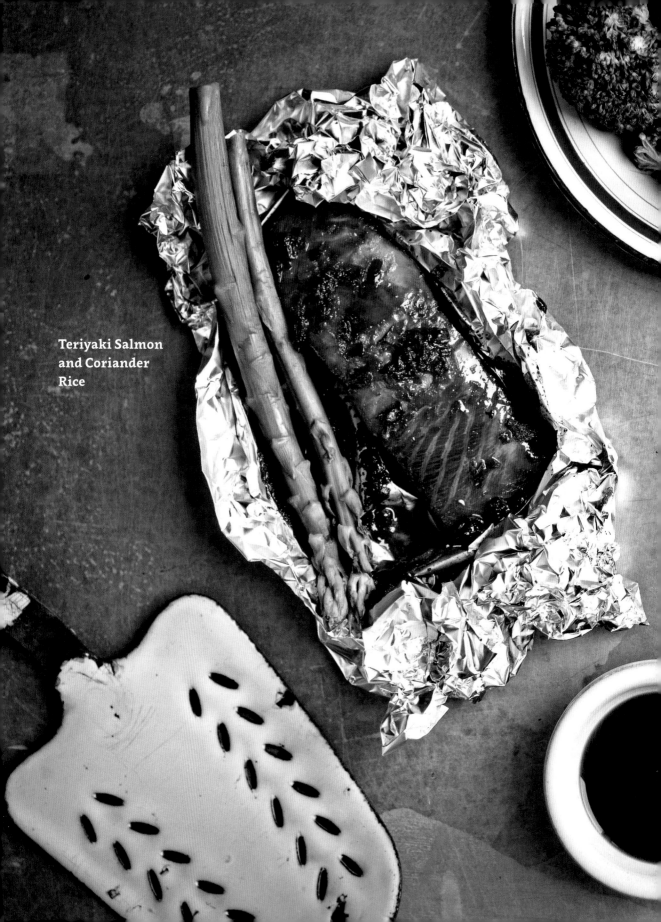

Teriyaki Salmon
and Coriander
Rice

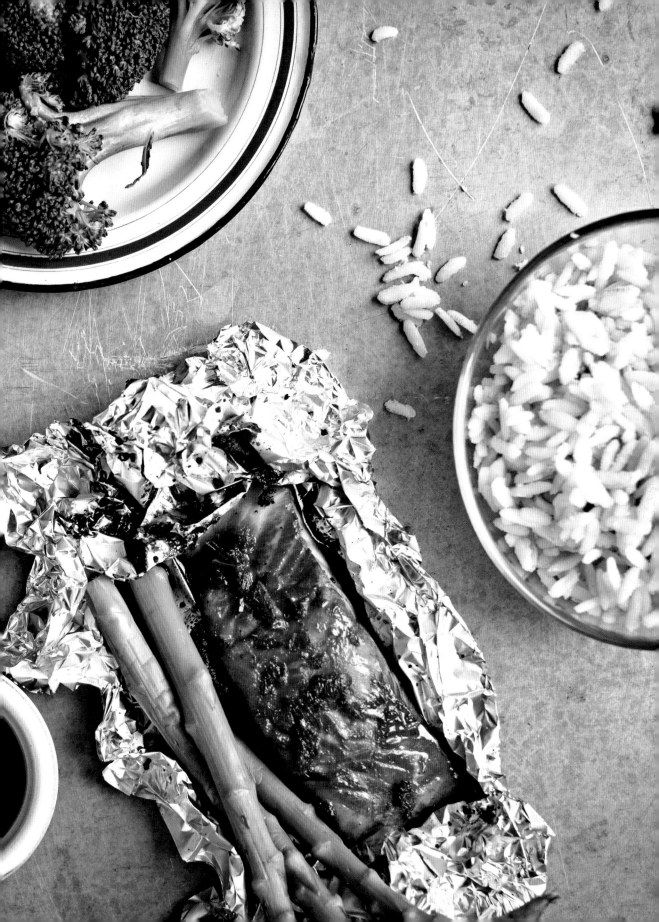

# CHILLI SALMON NOODLE BOWL

Store salmon fillets in the freezer to ensure that you always have a healthy option that can be made quickly. **Serves 2**

2 × 120 g salmon fillets
1 small red chilli pepper, finely
    chopped
1 tbsp rice vinegar
1 tbsp reduced-sodium soy sauce
2 tsp grated ginger
$^1/_2$ bunch of coriander, chopped
100 g wholewheat noodles
200 g mangetout
2 carrots, sliced
2 tbsp teriyaki sauce

**Calories:**
495

› Preheat the oven to 190°C/375°F/gas 5.
› Line a baking tray with parchment paper and put the salmon on it, skin side down.
› In a bowl, mix the chilli, rice vinegar, soy sauce, ginger and coriander, and spoon the sauce over the salmon.
› Roast the salmon in the oven for 15–20 minutes until cooked through.
› Put the noodles in a pot with water. Bring to the boil, reduce and simmer until cooked.
› In a large pan, or wok, add 1 tablespoon of water, mangetout and carrots, and cook until tender but still crisp.
› Stir in the teriyaki sauce, then add the cooked noodles and mix all together.
› Place on two plates and top with the salmon.

# INDIAN FISH CURRY

› Place the rice in a pot of water. Bring to the boil, then reduce the heat and simmer until light and fluffy.
› Place the oil in a large pan over a medium to high heat. Add the onion and cook for 7–10 minutes, until softened and starting to go light brown.
› Add the garlic and tomatoes, and cook for a further 2 minutes.
› Now add the curry paste, coconut milk and peppers, and bring to the boil.
› Reduce the heat to a simmer, add the fish and cook gently for 10–12 minutes, or until the fish is cooked through.
› Place the cooked rice on two plates and serve with the curry mixture. Top with chopped coriander.

Mix up this recipe by adding scallops or prawns instead of cod. **Serves 2**

60 g wholegrain rice
1 tsp rapeseed oil
1 large onion, chopped
1 clove of garlic, finely chopped
200 g tinned chopped tomatoes
1 tbsp curry paste
400 ml light coconut milk
1 red pepper, deseeded
   and chopped
1 yellow pepper, deseeded
   and  chopped
300 g white fish (cod, haddock,
   monkfish), cut into 4-cm chunks
$^1/_2$ bunch of coriander, chopped

**Calories:**
539

# FISH CAKES AND SALAD

Make these into finger shapes and this becomes a great option as a first food for the little ones in the house.

**Serves 2**

200 g potatoes, peeled and chopped
20 ml low-fat milk
2 tsp rapeseed oil
1/2 onion, finely chopped
250 g mixed fish pieces (salmon, white fish, smoked white fish)
40 g butternut squash, peeled and chopped
1 stick of celery, sliced
1 tbsp dill, stemmed
pinch of salt and pepper
1 egg
50 g breadcrumbs
2 tsp sweet chilli sauce

FOR THE SIDE SALAD:
50 g spinach
100 g cherry tomatoes, halved
30 g black-eyed beans
50 g sweetcorn

**Calories:**
510

› Preheat the oven to 220°C/425°F/gas 7.
› Place the potatoes in a pot of water. Bring to the boil, reduce the heat and simmer until tender.
› Drain the potatoes, add the milk and mash. Set aside.
› Place 1 teaspoon of oil in a pan over a medium heat. Add the onion and cook until soft. Remove and place in a bowl.
› To the same pan, add another teaspoon of oil. Then add the fish pieces and stir gently until cooked through – try to keep the fish in chunks.
› Steam the squash and celery until soft.
› Using a hand blender or a food processor, blend the squash, celery and onion until smooth.
› In a large bowl, combine the potatoes, dill and squash purée. Then mix in the fish.
› Season with salt and pepper, if liked.
› Beat the egg in a bowl and place the breadcrumbs in another bowl.
› Divide the fish cake mixture into six circular shapes about 2.5 cm thick.
› Dip each fish cake in egg and then into the breadcrumbs, and place on an oiled baking tray.
› Bake in the oven for 20 minutes, or until golden.
› Combine all the ingredients for the side salad in a bowl. Serve the fish cakes with the side salad and sweet chilli sauce.

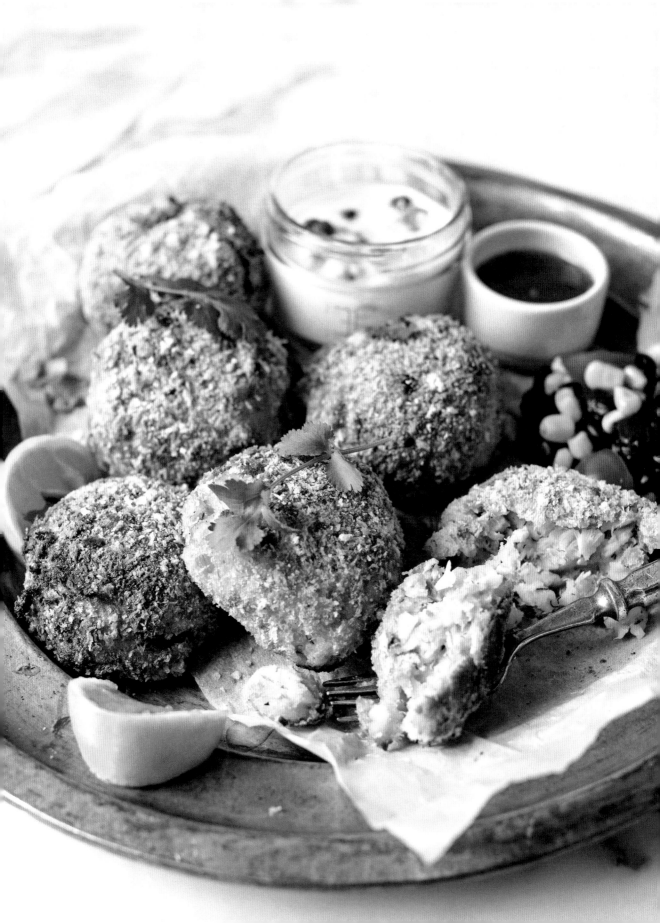

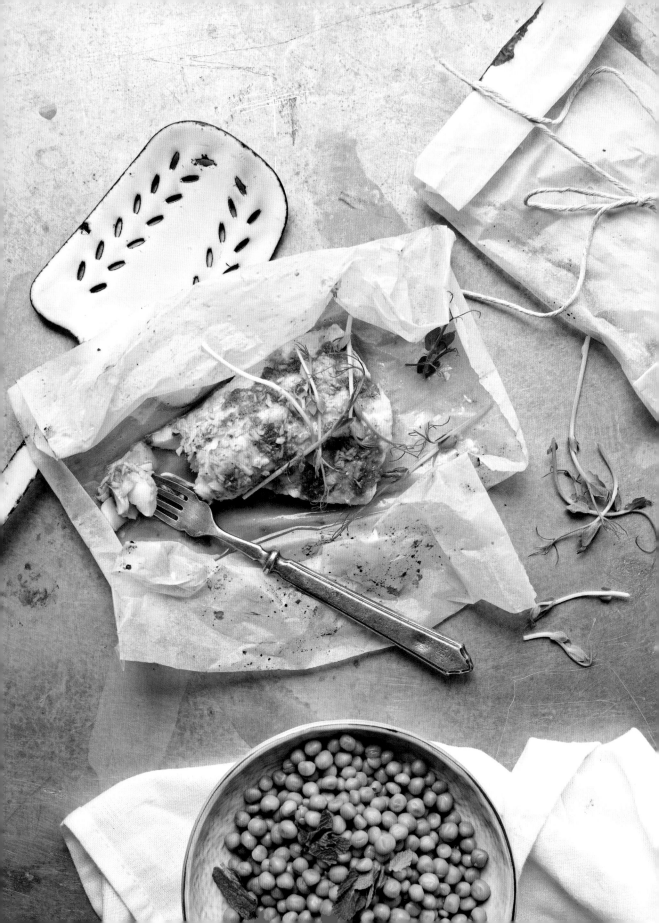

# CURRY COCONUT FISH PARCEL

› Preheat the oven to 200°C/400°F/gas 6.
› Tear off 2 large pieces of tinfoil, double them and place a fish fillet in the centre of each one.
› Spread the curry paste over each fillet.
› Combine the coconut, lime zest and juice, and soy sauce, and divide between each fillet.
› Bring up the sides of the foil and scrunch the edges and sides together to make 2 sealed parcels.
› Place the parcels on a baking tray and bake for 10–15 minutes until fully cooked.
› Place the rice in a pot of boiling water and cook until light and fluffy.
› Steam the peas.
› Serve each piece of fish on a bed of rice. Drizzle with sweet chilli sauce and add peas to the side.
› Garnish with sliced red chilli pepper.

Invest in good-quality curry paste from an Asian supermarket – it makes a big difference to the flavour. **Serves 2**

2 × 150 g white fish fillets (cod, haddock, monkfish)
2 tsp curry paste
1 tsp desiccated coconut
zest and juice of 1 lime
1 tsp reduced-sodium soy sauce
300 g frozen peas
100 g wholegrain rice
2 tbsp sweet chilli sauce
1 red chilli pepper, finely sliced

**Calories:**
505

The 'other white meat', as it's often referred to, unprocessed pork loin and pork steak are great low-fat protein options. It also adds a bit of variety to the week.

# PORK
# PORK TENDERLOIN WITH ORANGE MARINADE

I love this pork option as a change from a traditional roast at the weekend. For added flavour, you can marinate the pork overnight. This can be cooked in a slow cooker on low for 8 hours. **Serves 4**

240 ml orange juice
120 ml reduced-sodium soy sauce
2 tbsp balsamic vinegar
2–3 tbsp Dijon mustard
dash of hot sauce
4 cloves of garlic, crushed
500 g pork steak
1 turnip, peeled and chopped
3 carrots, chopped
800 g baby potatoes

**Calories:**
404

› Preheat the oven to 175°C/350°F/gas 4.
› Combine the juice, soy sauce, vinegar, mustard, hot sauce and garlic in an ovenproof dish.
› Add the pork steak to the marinade and place in the oven to cook for an hour.
› Add the turnip and carrots to a pot of water, bring to the boil, then turn down the heat and simmer until soft. Drain the vegetables and mash together.
› Add the potatoes to a large pot of cold water and bring to the boil. Turn down the heat and simmer until soft. Drain off the water.
› Remove the pork from the oven and cut into 100 g servings per person.
› Divide the vegetables and potatoes between plates and serve hot.

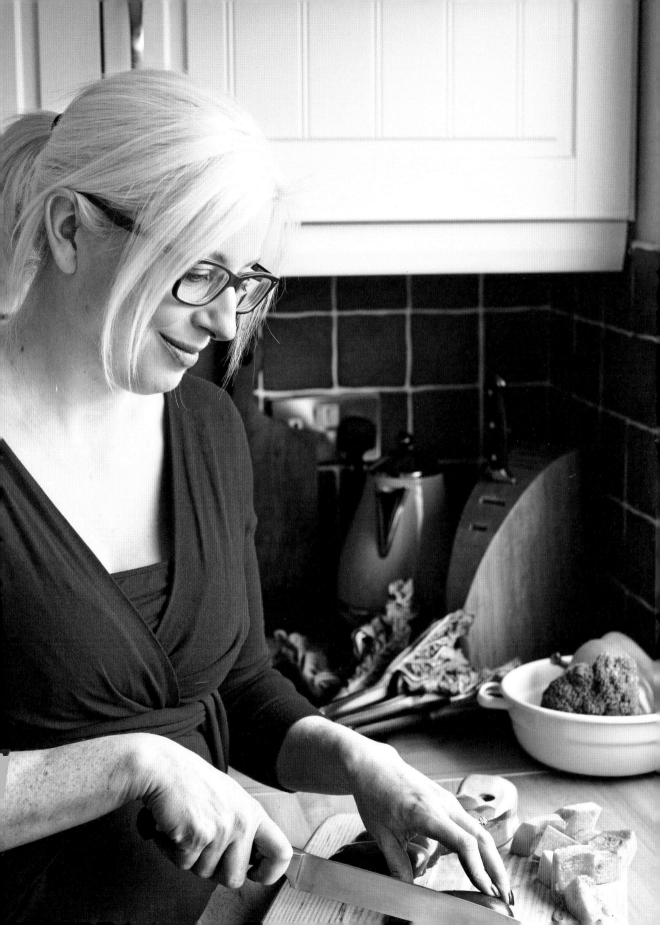

# SPICY PORK AND CARROT STIR-FRY

Quick and easy – I love it because it is such a simple but tasty recipe.

**Serves 2**

2 pork loin chops, cut into strips with fat removed
2 cloves of garlic, finely chopped
1 tbsp reduced-sodium soy sauce
1½ tsp cumin
1 red chilli pepper, finely chopped
100 g wholegrain rice
1 tbsp rapeseed oil
1 onion, sliced
2 carrots, chopped
2 tbsp chopped coriander

**Calories:**
554

› Combine the pork, garlic, soy sauce, cumin and chilli pepper in a bowl.
› Put the wholegrain rice into a pot of boiling water and cook until light and fluffy.
› In a wok, heat the oil. Add the onion and carrots, and cook until crisp.
› Add the pork mixture and cook until browned, about 2 minutes. Stir until cooked through.
› Serve with the rice and garnish with the coriander.

# SWEET AND SOUR PORK

› In a medium bowl, beat the egg white with a fork until slightly frothy.
› Beat in the five-spice powder, 1 tablespoon of cornflour, flour and pepper.
› Stir in the pork so that each piece is coated.
› To make the sauce, mix the soy sauce, vinegar, tomato purée, blended cornflour and water, and stock, and set aside.
› Put the rice in a pot of boiling water and cook until light and fluffy.
› Heat the oil in a wok on a medium to high heat.
› Add the pork strips and stir-fry for about 5 minutes, or until the pork is no longer pink.
› Then add the garlic, ginger, spring onions, pepper and carrot, and stir-fry for 2–4 minutes.
› Pour in the sauce and continue to cook until the vegetables are tender and the pork is cooked through.
› Serve the rice and top with the sweet and sour pork.

Make the sweet and sour sauce ahead of time to make this a quick mid-week option. **Serves 2**

1 egg white
$1/4$ tsp five-spice powder
1 tbsp cornflour
$1^1/2$ tsp flour
1 tsp pepper
2 pork loin chops, cut into strips
1 tsp reduced-sodium soy sauce
1 tbsp rice wine vinegar
1 tsp tomato purée
1 tsp cornflour blended with
    1 tsp water
175 ml reduced-sodium vegetable stock
80 g wholegrain rice
1 tbsp rapeseed oil
2 cloves of garlic, finely chopped
2 tsp ginger, finely chopped
2 spring onions, chopped
1 red pepper, deseeded and chopped
1 carrot, chopped

**Calories:**
510

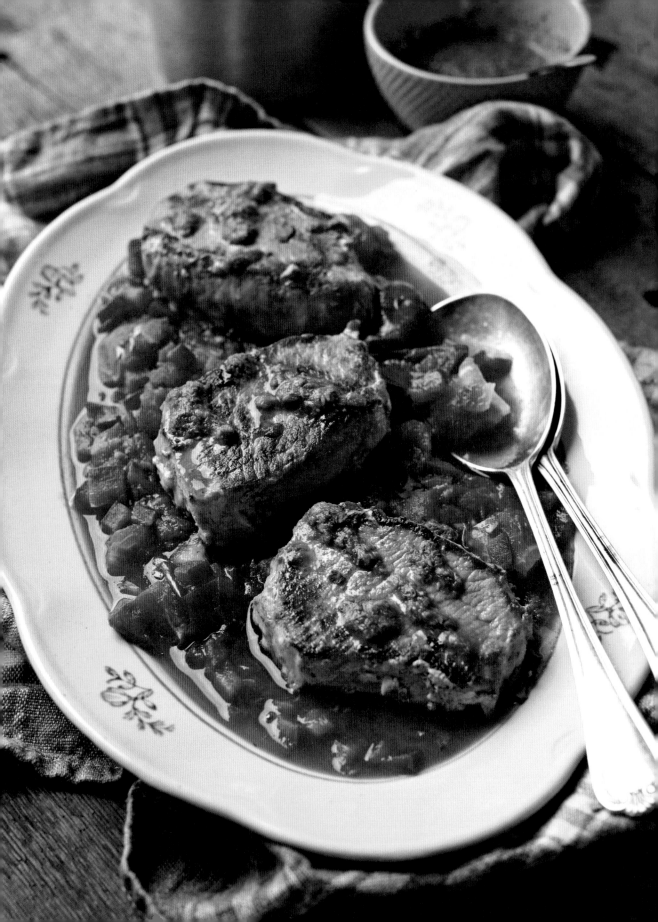

# PORK MEDALLIONS WITH SUPER GREEN SAUCE

› To make the super green sauce, combine the capers, coriander, spring onions, 1 teaspoon of oil and 1 ½ teaspoons of water in a food processor or hand blender.
› Remove all the fat from the pork chops.
› Add 2 teaspoons of oil to a pan over a medium to high heat and add the pork chops. Cover and cook on each side until cooked through.
› Add the tomatoes and pepper, and cook until slightly softened.
› Place the potatoes in a pot and add water. Bring to the boil, then reduce the heat and simmer until tender. Drain the potatoes, add milk and mash. Season with salt and pepper, if liked.
› Serve the pork chops with the tomatoes and peppers, drizzle with the super green sauce and finish with the mashed potatoes.

I love the flavour coriander brings to this meal. **Serves 2**

2 tbsp capers
bunch of coriander, chopped
bunch of spring onions
3 tsp olive oil
300 g pork loin chops
8 tomatoes or 300 g tinned
   chopped tomatoes
1 red pepper, deseeded
   and chopped
300 g potatoes, peeled
50 ml low-fat milk
pinch of salt and pepper

**Calories:**
436

# PORK WITH SPROUTS

Sprouts are not just for Christmas!
**Serves 2**

1¹/₂ tsp cornflour
2¹/₂ tbsp reduced-sodium
    soy sauce
300 g pork loin chops, cut into
    5-cm medallions
1 tbsp balsamic vinegar
1¹/₂ tsp rice wine
2 tsp rapeseed oil
400 g Brussels sprouts, trimmed
    and halved
1 tbsp grated ginger
1 clove of garlic, finely sliced
¹/₄ tsp chilli flakes
80 g wholegrain rice

**Calories:**
511

› In a bowl, mix the cornflour with 1 ½ tablespoons of soy sauce. Add the pork medallions and coat with the mixture.
› In a separate bowl, combine the remaining soy sauce, vinegar, rice wine and 1 tablespoon of water.
› Heat the oil in a pan and add the sprouts. Cook over a high heat for 5 minutes. To provide a shot of steam, add water.
› Add the ginger, garlic and chilli flakes.
› Then add the coated pork and cook for 5 minutes until golden but not completely cooked through.
› Add the soy sauce mixture and simmer until the pork is cooked through.
› Put the rice in a pot of boiling water and cook until light and fluffy.
› Serve the pork and Brussels sprouts sauce on a bed of rice.

# PORK STEAK WITH PEPPERS AND CREAMY POLENTA

› Preheat the oven to 220°C/425°F/gas 7.
› Put 1 teaspoon of oil into an ovenproof dish. Add the pork steak and season with salt and pepper, if liked.
› Cover with tinfoil, and place in the oven and bake for 45 minutes, or until cooked through.
› Combine 100 ml of chicken stock, cornflour and vinegar in a small bowl. Pour into a pot and bring to the boil. Cook for about 2 minutes, or until the sauce is slightly thickened.
› Add 1 teaspoon of oil to a pan and put on a medium to high heat.
› Add the thyme, garlic and peppers, and cook until the peppers are crisp.
› In a pot, bring the milk and remaining chicken stock to a simmer.
› Gradually add the polenta, stirring constantly with a whisk. Reduce the heat and simmer for 10 minutes, until the liquid is completely absorbed.
› Serve the pork with the peppers and polenta.

Polenta is a great gluten-free carbohydrate option at dinner.

**Serves 4**

2 tsp rapeseed oil
455 g pork steak
pinch of salt and pepper
500 ml reduced-sodium chicken stock
1 tsp cornflour
1 tsp cider vinegar
2 tsp chopped thyme
2 cloves of garlic, crushed
1 red pepper, deseeded and chopped
1 green pepper, deseeded and chopped
1 yellow pepper, deseeded and chopped
400 ml low-fat milk
120 g polenta

**Calories:**
367

Ireland has a love affair with chicken. Chicken is a quick and easy protein choice, but make sure it doesn't take over from other protein options. Although chicken is often looked on as a cheap option, as with everything in life, you get what you pay for. When possible, choose local, outdoor-reared/free-range chicken for the best quality.

# POULTRY
# CHICKEN AND CHORIZO PASTA BAKE

A great family favourite!
## Serves 4

200 g wholewheat penne pasta
1 courgette, chopped
1 green pepper, deseeded
    and chopped
1 sweet pointer pepper, deseeded
    and chopped
350 g chicken breast, chopped into
    2.5 cm pieces
2 tbsp sun-dried tomato pesto
90 g sun-dried tomatoes, chopped
2 × 400 g tins chopped tomatoes
bunch of basil, chopped, or 3 tsp
    dried basil
100 g chorizo, sliced

## Calories:
551

› Preheat the oven to 200°C/400°F/gas 6.
› Put the penne pasta in a pot with plenty of water and cook for about 10 minutes until slightly underdone.
› Place all the vegetables in an ovenproof dish. Add the chicken, pesto, sun-dried tomatoes, chopped tomatoes, basil and chorizo. Stir in the cooked pasta.
› Cover and place in the oven for 45–60 minutes until the chicken is cooked through.
› Remove the cover and cook for a further 10 minutes for a crispy top.

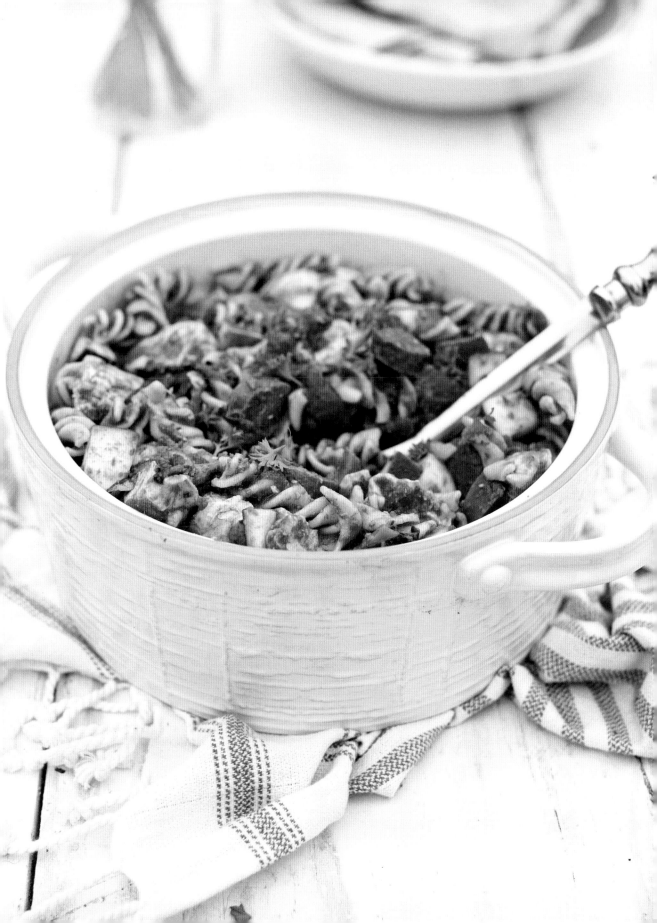

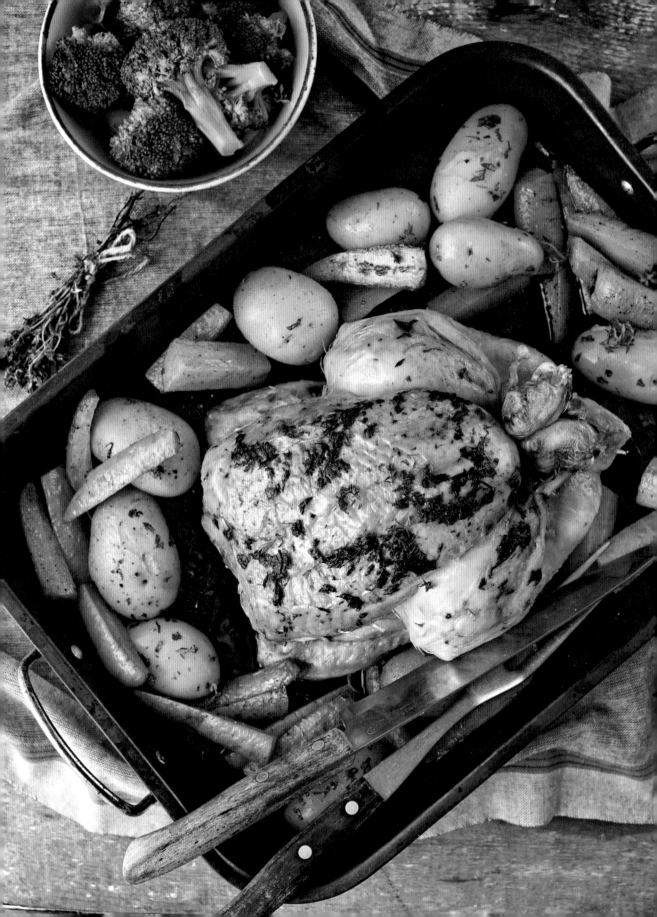

# HERBY
# ROAST CHICKEN

› Preheat the oven to 140°C/275°F/gas 1.
› Using a rolling pin, roughly bash the garlic cloves. Then place in a large food bag with the rosemary, thyme, sage, lemon zest and oil. (You can leave this to marinate overnight for added flavour.)
› Rub the marinade into the chicken, inside and out.
› Put the vegetables (except the potatoes) in a large roasting dish and top with the chicken.
› Scatter any remaining herbs and garlic from the marinade over and around and inside the chicken.
› Cut the discarded lemon in half and stuff inside the chicken, along with the rosemary.
› Rub the skin of the chicken all over with butter. Cover with tinfoil and cook for 3 hours.
› Add the halved potatoes to a large pot of cold water and boil for 10–12 minutes.
› When cooked, drain the potatoes and shake them in the pot with the lid still on.
› Put 2 teaspoons of rapeseed oil in an ovenproof dish and add the potatoes. Sprinkle 1 teaspoon of oil on top of the potatoes and place in the oven for 30–45 minutes.
› Remove the foil from the chicken and continue cooking for a further 1 hour or until the chicken is cooked and the juices run clear. Increase the oven to 220°C/425°F/gas 7 and roast for 25–30 minutes until the skin is crisp.
› Lift the chicken from the dish and place on a plate to rest, before serving with the vegetables and potatoes.

Yes, this really does say cook for 4 ½ hours – but the taste justifies the effort, I promise!

**Serves 4 (with leftovers)**

1 bulb of garlic, cloves separated
bunch each of rosemary, thyme, and sage
zest of 1 lemon
6 tsp rapeseed oil
1 medium-sized whole chicken (200 g cooked chicken meat per serving)
2 carrots, chopped
2 parsnips, chopped
1 small turnip, peeled and chopped
1 red onion, chopped
1 tbsp butter
500 g potatoes, peeled and halved

**Calories:**
403

# CHICKEN AND LOADED-VEGETABLE BAKE

A great option for the whole family.

**Serves 4**

3 tbsp butter
30 g flour
4 chicken fillets
1 red onion, chopped
3 carrots, chopped
2 sticks of celery, chopped
1 small head of cauliflower,
   florets  halved
bunch of parsley, chopped
1 bay leaf
a few black peppercorns
300 ml low-fat milk
1 large head of broccoli, chopped
50 g breadcrumbs
500 g potatoes, peeled chopped

**Calories:**
543

› Preheat the oven to 180°C/350°F/gas 4.
› Combine 2 tablespoons of butter and flour.
› Place the chicken, onion, carrots, celery, cauliflower, parsley, bay leaf, peppercorns, and enough water to cover, in a pot and slowly bring to the boil.
› Reduce the heat and simmer until the chicken is cooked, about 20–30 minutes.
› Remove the chicken fillets from the pot and leave to cool.
› Strain the cooking liquid into a saucepan and bring to the boil. Add the milk, then turn down the heat and simmer for 2–3 minutes.
› Return to the boil and beat in the butter and flour mixture, a small amount at a time, until the sauce thickens, then remove from the heat.
› Place the cooked vegetables (onion, carrots, celery and cauliflower) in a bowl and blend with a hand blender or food processor until smooth.
› Meanwhile, steam the broccoli and chop the chicken fillets into bite-sized chunks.
› Melt the remaining butter and combine with the breadcrumbs.
› Combine the chicken, broccoli, potatoes and vegetable sauce in an ovenproof dish.
› Cover with the breadcrumb mixture.
› Bake in the oven for 20–30 minutes until golden on top.

# MANGO CHICKEN

> - Preheat the oven to 200°C/400°F/gas 6.
> - Mix the mango chutney, natural yogurt and wholegrain mustard in a bowl.
> - Put 1 teaspoon of oil and the chicken in an ovenproof dish lined with tinfoil.
> - Pour the chutney mixture on top of the chicken, then cover and place in the oven for 20 minutes until cooked through.
> - Steam the broccoli.
> - Fill a pot with water and boil the sweet potato for 10–12 minutes. Remove from the water and chop into large chunks.
> - Put 1 teaspoon of oil in a baking dish, add the chopped sweet potato and sprinkle 1 teaspoon of oil over the chunks and cook for 20–30 minutes.
> - Serve the mango chicken, broccoli and roasted sweet potato on two plates.

This can be a great option for the younger members of the family – cut the potatoes and chicken into strips to make this a great finger food meal. **Serves 2**

2 tbsp mango chutney
30 g natural yogurt (3% fat)
2 tbsp wholegrain mustard
3 tsp rapeseed oil
2 chicken fillets
300 g broccoli florets
400 g sweet potato, peeled

**Calories:**
548

# CHICKEN AND GINGER CURRY

To add more flavour to this meal, you can add 1 teaspoon each of coriander seeds, cumin seeds and mustard seeds to the pot before adding the rice. **Serves 2**

1 tbsp rapeseed oil
350 g chicken breast, chopped into 2.5 cm pieces
2 cloves of garlic, finely chopped
2 tbsp grated or easy ginger
1 large onion, chopped
2 carrots, chopped
½ small turnip, peeled and chopped
240 ml reduced-sodium chicken stock
1–2 tbsp curry paste
100 g wholegrain rice

**Calories:**
553

› Heat the oil in a large skillet, or pan, on a medium to high heat.
› Add the chicken and cook until lightly brown.
› Add the garlic, ginger, onion, carrots and turnip to the skillet, and sauté together for a further 5 minutes.
› Add the chicken stock and curry paste, and simmer for 5–10 minutes.
› For spicy rice, toast the coriander, cumin and mustard seeds in a medium-sized saucepan. When the seeds pop and become fragrant, add water and bring to the boil. Add the rice and prepare as usual.
› When cooked, divide the rice between two plates and serve the chicken and ginger curry on top.

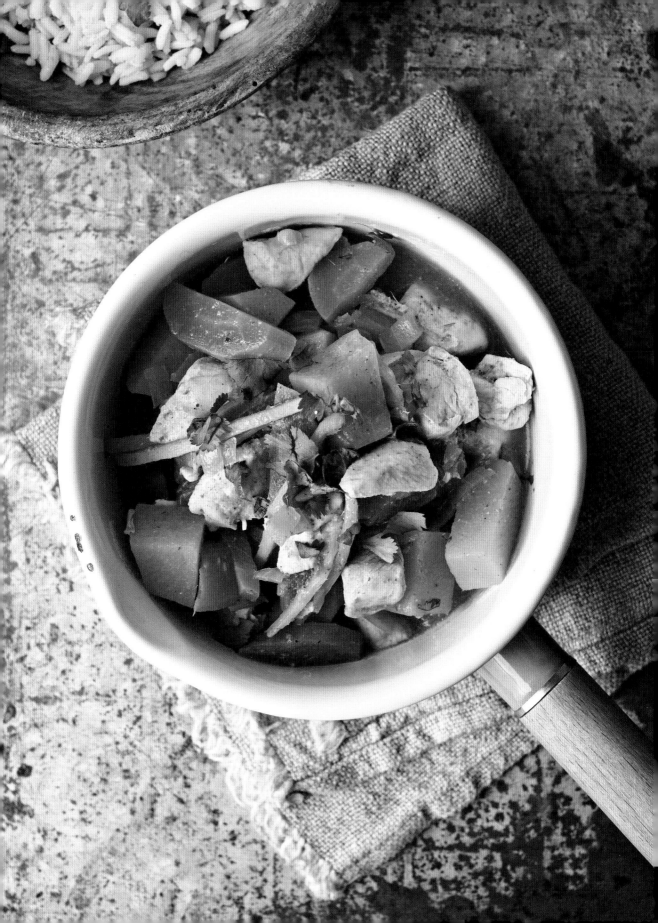

# CHICKEN FAJITAS

Make sure to have a stash of fajita spice mix (page 210) in the cupboard to make this option an easy one. **Serves 2**

250 g chicken breast, cut into strips
2 tbsp fajita spice mix (page 210)
2 tsp rapeseed oil
1 red pepper, deseeded
    and chopped
1 green pepper, deseeded
    and chopped
1 red onion, chopped
juice of 1 lime
dash of hot sauce
dash of Worcestershire sauce
2 wholewheat wraps
30 g salsa
2 tbsp natural yogurt (3% fat)

FOR THE SIDE SALAD:
100 g butterhead lettuce
¹/₂ cucumber, sliced
2 tomatoes, sliced

**Calories:**
532

› Combine the chicken strips with the fajita spice mix.
› Put the oil in a large skillet, or pan, on a medium to high heat.
› Add the chicken and cook for 3–5 minutes until lightly brown.
› Add the chopped vegetables along with the lime juice, hot sauce and Worcestershire sauce.
› Cook for a further 15 minutes on a medium heat.
› Serve with a wholewheat wrap, salsa, natural yogurt and a side salad.

# CHICKEN QUESADILLAS AND SALAD

› Heat 2 teaspoons of oil in a pan on a medium to high heat.
› Add the chicken strips and sauté until cooked through, or use leftover roast chicken.
› Remove the chicken and set aside.
› Heat 1 teaspoon of oil in the same pan, on a medium heat, and add a wholewheat wrap and heat through.
› Spread orange marmalade on the wholewheat wrap in the pan, followed by the chicken, kidney beans, roasted peppers, coriander and pinch of salt to season.
› Top with another wholewheat wrap. Cook for 2–3 minutes until the bottom wrap is golden.
› To toast the top wrap, place under a grill on medium heat.
› Serve with the natural yogurt and a side salad.

This can be a quick Monday meal if using leftovers from a roast at the weekend. **Serves 2**

3 tsp rapeseed oil
250 g chicken breast, cut into strips
2 wholewheat wraps
3 tsp orange marmalade
4 tbsp kidney beans
2 roasted peppers (from a jar is fine)
2 tbsp chopped or 1 tbsp dried coriander
pinch of salt
dash of hot sauce (optional)
30 g natural yogurt (3% fat)

FOR THE SIDE SALAD:
50 g salad leaves
$1/2$ cucumber, sliced
2 tomatoes, sliced

**Calories:**
550

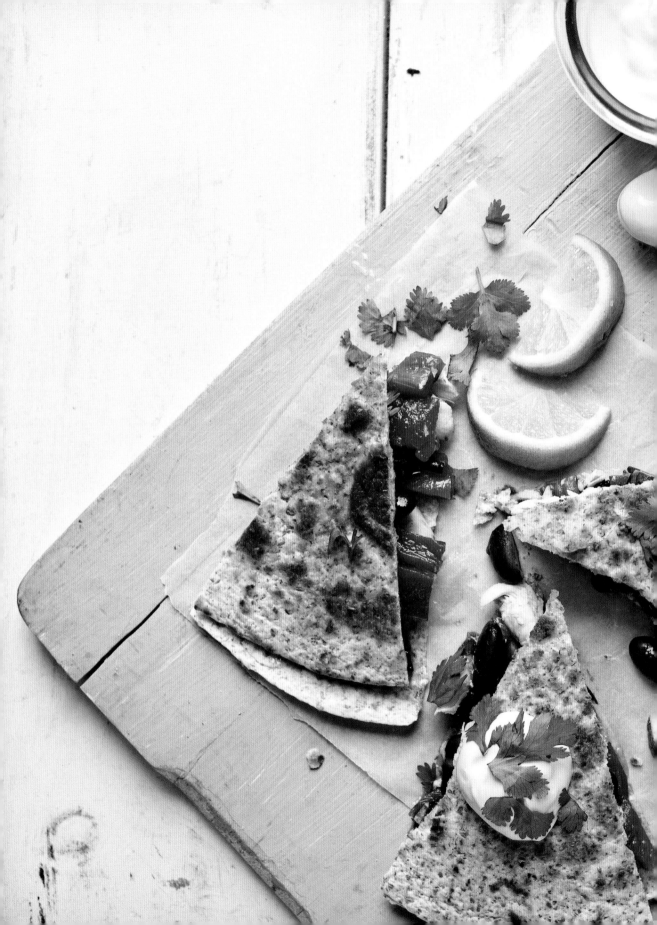

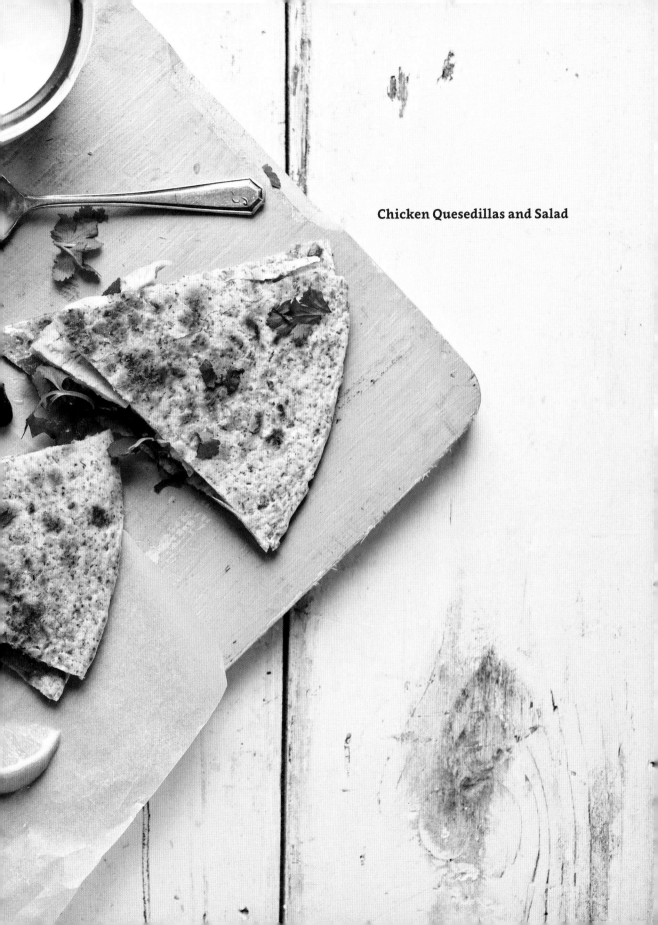

Chicken Quesedillas and Salad

# SPANISH CHICKEN

A one-pot meal – who doesn't love that?! A great option for the slow cooker. **Serves 2**

10 g flour
2 tsp paprika
2 tsp smoked paprika
½ tsp pepper
250 g chicken breast, cut into
    bite-sized pieces
3 tsp rapeseed oil
2 cloves of garlic, crushed
1 onion, chopped
1 yellow pepper, deseeded and cut
    into chunks
1 green pepper, deseeded and cut
    into chunks
1 red pepper, deseeded and cut
    into chunks
500 ml reduced-sodium
    chicken stock
2 tbsp tomato purée
100 g wholegrain rice
1 tbsp chopped parsley

**Calories:**
547

› In a bowl, mix the flour, paprika, smoked paprika and pepper. Add the chicken and mix so that the chicken is coated.
› Add 2 teaspoons of oil to a pot on a medium to high heat.
› Add the coated chicken and cook for 3–4 minutes, then remove and set aside.
› Put the remaining oil into the same pot with the garlic and onion, and sauté for 2–3 minutes. Then add the peppers for a further 5 minutes.
› Pour in the stock, tomato purée and raw rice.
› Return the chicken, cover and simmer for 20–30 minutes until the chicken is completely cooked.
› Be sure to stir regularly to prevent the rice catching at the bottom of the pot.
› Garnish with parsley and serve hot.

# STUFFED CHICKEN WITH LEMON, CAPERS AND CHILLI

› Preheat the oven to 200°C/400°F/gas 6.
› Cut a slit in the side of each chicken fillet and use your finger to make a pocket.
› Mix half the lemon zest, Parmesan, capers and chilli flakes.
› Place a slice of mozzarella and some of the mixture into the pocket of each chicken fillet and secure with a cocktail stick.
› Put the chicken in an ovenproof dish and drizzle with half the oil. Bake for 15–20 minutes until cooked through.
› Meanwhile, heat the remaining oil in a pot over a medium heat. Add the garlic and cook for 1–2 minutes – be careful not to burn it.
› Add the tomatoes and simmer for 10 minutes until the sauce has thickened slightly.
› Place the potatoes in a pot of boiling water and simmer until cooked. Steam the broccoli.
› Spoon the tomato mixture onto each plate and top with the chicken.
› Serve with the potatoes and broccoli.

This meal takes a while to prepare, so it is best to make it when you have a little more time on your hands. Stuff the chicken fillets ahead of time to make this a quick option for mid-week. **Serves 2**

2 chicken fillets
30 g mozzarella cheese, sliced
zest of 1 lemon
1 tbsp Parmesan, grated
1 tsp capers
1 tsp chilli flakes
$1^1/_2$ tbsp rapeseed oil
2 cloves of garlic, finely chopped
1 × 400 g tin chopped tomatoes
200 g potatoes
200 g broccoli florets

**Calories:**
452

# GRANNY BRID'S CHICKEN

I still don't think I cook this as well as my mother-in-law – but it always goes down a treat! **Serves 2**

300 g potatoes, peeled and cut into 2.5 cm cubes

3 tsp olive oil

30 g chorizo, cut into cubes

200 g roasted red peppers (from a jar is okay)

350 g chicken breast, cut into 2.5 cm strips

1 tsp paprika

1 tsp smoked paprika

2 tbsp cooking cream

**Calories:**
492

› Preheat the oven to 220°C/425°F/gas 7.
› Put the potato cubes in a pot of water and boil until partly cooked. Then drain.
› Oil a baking tray with 1 teaspoon of oil and spread the potatoes on the tray. Drizzle 1 teaspoon of oil over the potato cubes.
› Place in the oven and cook for 20–30 minutes until brown and crispy on the outside.
› Slice the peppers into strips and place in a bowl.
› Heat 1 teaspoon of oil in a deep pan over a medium to high heat. Add the chorizo cubes and stir for a few minutes to stop them burning.
› Spoon the peppers into the pan.
› Add the chicken, stirring occasionally, until the chicken goes a white or light brown colour.
› Scatter the paprika and smoked paprika into the pan, coating the chicken.
› Add the cream and cook until the chicken is cooked through.

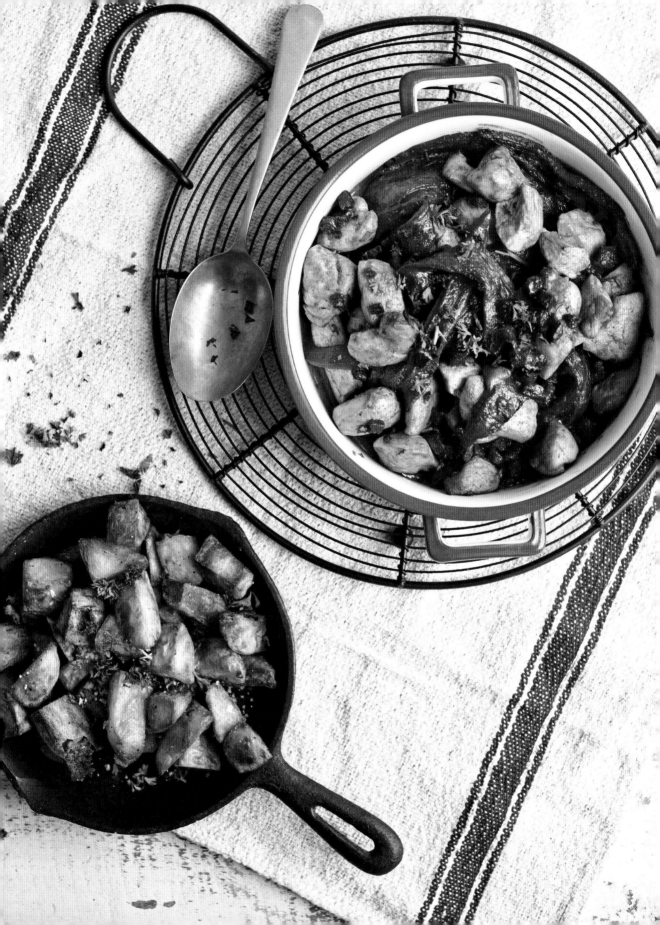

# TEX MEX CHICKEN AND WHOLEWHEAT NOODLES

Any leftover chicken and vegetables from this meal would be great in a wrap for lunch the following day.

**Serves 2**

100 g wholewheat noodles
3 tsp olive oil
300 g chicken breast, cut into strips
1 tsp chilli powder (more if you like it spicy!)
$1/2$ onion, chopped
1 green pepper, deseeded and chopped
1 red pepper, deseeded and chopped
3 tbsp water
1 × 400 g tin chopped tomatoes
15 g natural yogurt (3% fat)
2 tsp chopped coriander

**Calories:**
509

› Place the noodles in a pot of water and bring to the boil, then simmer until cooked.
› Place a deep pan over a medium to high heat and add 2 teaspoons of oil.
› Add the chicken and chilli powder, stirring occasionally, until the chicken is cooked through. Transfer to a bowl.
› Add the remaining oil, onion, peppers and water to the pan and reduce the heat. Continue stirring until the vegetables soften.
› Increase the heat to medium, then add the tomatoes, cooked noodles and chicken.
› Serve topped with natural yogurt and chopped coriander.

# ROAST BASIL CHICKEN

- › Preheat the oven to 220°C/425°F/gas 7.
- › Place the basil in a pot of water, bring to the boil and let it boil for just 30 seconds. Then drain and rinse the basil under cold water.
- › Put the basil, butter, garlic, lemon zest and salt, if liked, in a food processor (or use a hand processor) and blend to a smooth purée.
- › Place the chicken in a baking dish and rub with half of the basil butter mixture, making sure to place some under the skin as well.
- › Cook in the oven for 1 ½ –2 hours until cooked through.
- › Add the potatoes to a saucepan of water, and bring to the boil. Reduce the heat and simmer until tender.
- › Steam the broccoli and carrots.
- › Drain the potatoes and add the remaining basil butter.
- › Serve the chicken (without skin), and add vegetables and potatoes to each plate.

The basil adds a fresh twist to this Sunday roast. **Serves 4**

bunch of basil
1 tbsp butter
1 clove of garlic, grated
zest of 1 lemon
pinch of salt
1 medium-sized whole chicken
   (200 g cooked meat per serving)
300 g baby potatoes
150 g broccoli florets
300 g carrots, chopped

**Calories:**
439

# FIVE-SPICE CHICKEN

You can marinate the chicken overnight in the spice mixture to add extra flavour to this recipe.

**Serves 2**

2 tbsp five-spice powder
1 tsp garlic powder
¹/₄ tsp chilli powder
2 tbsp reduced-sodium soy sauce
2 tsp rice vinegar
1 tbsp olive oil
350 g chicken breast
80 g wholegrain rice
300 g broccoli florets
3 tbsp chopped coriander

**Calories:**
476

› Preheat the oven to 220°C/425°F/gas 7.
› In a large bowl, mix the five-spice, garlic and chilli powders. Add the soy sauce and vinegar.
› Coat the chicken in this spicy sauce.
› Spread the oil on a baking tray and place the coated chicken on the tray.
› Cover the chicken with tinfoil and place in the oven for 30 minutes.
› Add rice to a pot of water and cook until light and fluffy.
› Steam the broccoli.
› After 30 minutes, remove the chicken from the oven and take off the tinfoil. Put back in the oven for a further 10 minutes, or until the chicken is cooked through.
› Serve and garnish with coriander.

# ROAST ITALIAN-STYLE SPICY CHICKEN

› Preheat the oven to 220°C/425°F/gas 7.
› In a bowl, add the rosemary, oregano, chilli peppers, lemon zest and juice, and tablespoon of pepper.
› Place the chicken in an ovenproof dish. Rub with the herb mixture, making sure to put some under the skin. Cover with tinfoil.
› Roast the chicken for 60 minutes. After 60 minutes, remove the tinfoil and cook for a further 30–45 minutes until the chicken is cooked through.
› Place the vegetables in a bowl and mix with 2 teaspoons of oil.
› Put the oiled vegetables on a baking tray, in a single layer. Roast for 20 minutes until tender.
› Place the potatoes in a large pot and cover with cold water. Bring to the boil and simmer for 10–15 minutes. Drain the potatoes.
› Place 1 teaspoon of oil in an ovenproof dish and add the potatoes. Sprinkle 1 teaspoon of oil on top of the potatoes and put in the oven for 30–45 minutes.
› Season with salt and pepper, as desired.

Use Golden Wonder potatoes to make lovely roast potatoes that are fluffy on the inside. **Serves 4**

1 tbsp chopped rosemary leaves
1 tbsp chopped oregano
2 chilli peppers, finely chopped
2 tsp lemon zest
1 tbsp lemon juice
1 tbsp pepper
1 medium-sized whole chicken (200 g of cooked meat per serving)
2 red peppers, deseeded and chopped
1 yellow pepper, deseeded and chopped
1 large onion, chopped
4 tsp rapeseed oil
400 g potatoes

**Calories:**
480

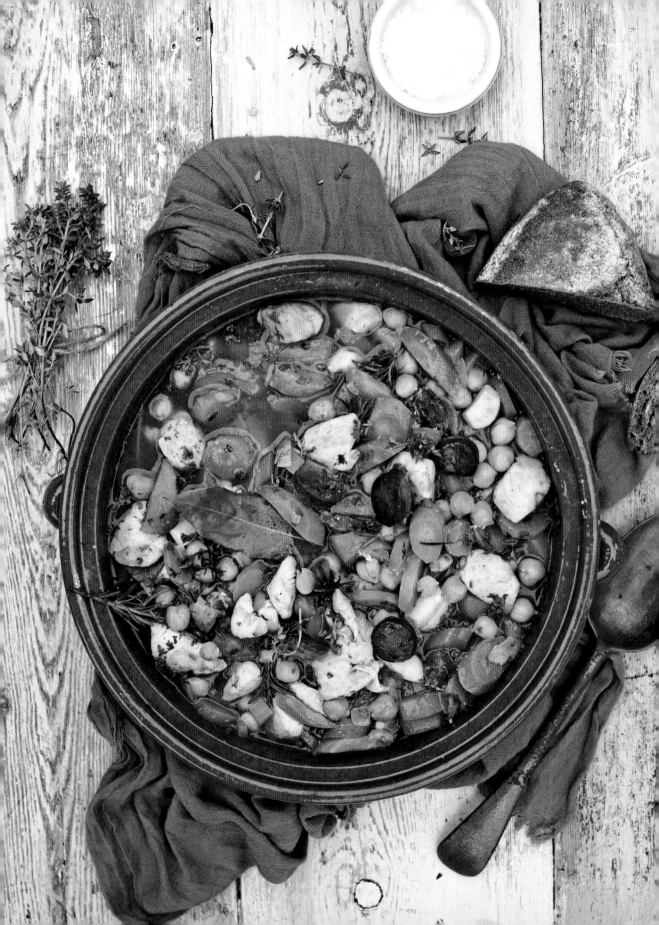

# SPANISH CHICKEN STEW WITH CHICKPEAS

› Preheat the oven to 200°C/400°F/gas 6.
› Heat the oil in a pan over a medium to high heat. Add the chicken and chorizo and cook until browned. Remove and add to a casserole dish.
› Turn the heat to low or medium. Add the onions to the pan and fry gently for 10 minutes until softened. Remove and add to the casserole dish.
› Add the garlic, chicken stock, saffron, bay leaves, rosemary, thyme, parsley, lemon zest, carrots and chickpeas to the casserole dish. Place in the oven, covered with a lid, for 15 minutes.
› Turn down oven to 180°C/350°F/gas 4 and cook for a further 30–45 minutes until the chicken and chickpeas are cooked through.
› Serve hot.

Chop the onions and potatoes ahead of time to make the preparation quicker. **Serves 4**

1 tbsp olive oil
350 g chicken breast, cut into bite-sized pieces
100 g chorizo, sliced
2 onions, finely chopped
1 bulb of garlic, cloves separated
500 ml reduced-sodium chicken stock
pinch of saffron
2 bay leaves
1 sprig of rosemary
2 sprigs of thyme
bunch of parsley, chopped
zest of $1/2$ lemon
6 carrots, chopped
300 g tinned chickpeas, drained and rinsed

**Calories:**
412

# CHICKEN PARMESAN

My take on chicken Parmesan – it brings back great memories of my time in America. **Serves 2**

100 g wholewheat pasta
340 g tomatoes, chopped
3 tsp rapeseed oil
1 clove of garlic, finely sliced
pinch of chilli flakes
2 chicken fillets
$\frac{1}{2}$ tsp dried oregano
20 g mozzarella cheese, sliced
1 tbsp Parmesan cheese, grated

**Calories:**
505

› Preheat the oven to 200°C/400°F/gas 6.
› Place the pasta in a pot of boiling water and simmer over a medium heat until cooked.
› Add the tomatoes and 1 teaspoon of oil to a medium-sized pot over a medium heat.
› Add the garlic and cook for about 1 minute, then add the chilli flakes. Bring to a simmer and cook for a further 8–10 minutes until the sauce thickens.
› Toss the chicken with the remaining oil and oregano.
› Put the chicken in an ovenproof baking dish and cover with tinfoil. Cook for 20–30 minutes until cooked through.
› Place the chicken on two plates, top with mozzarella and then tomato mixture. Sprinkle the Parmesan over the top. Serve with the pasta.

# GRILLED CHICKEN AND SWEETCORN SALAD WITH CHILLI CREAM DRESSING

› Combine the cream and chilli pepper in a saucepan and place on a low to medium heat, stirring occasionally. Simmer for about 5 minutes.
› In a bowl, drizzle the chicken and corn with 2 teaspoons of oil, and season with thyme, oregano, cumin, pepper and salt, if liked.
› Place 2 teaspoons of oil in a wok and heat over a medium heat. Add the chicken mixture, stirring occasionally until cooked through.
› Whisk together the lime juice, honey and 2 teaspoons of oil. Toss with the romaine lettuce and spinach.
› Place the salad leaves on a plate and top with the chicken, avocado and chilli cream dressing.

This is a lovely fresh dish – great for warm summer evenings! **Serves 1**

4 tbsp cooking cream
4 tsp chopped chilli peppers
2 x 100 g chicken breast, cut into bite-sized pieces
100 g sweetcorn
6 tsp olive oil
2 tsp chopped thyme
$^1/_2$ tsp dried oregano
$^1/_2$ tsp cumin
pinch of salt and pepper
juice of 1 lime
1 tsp honey
200 g romaine lettuce
100 g baby spinach
$^1/_2$ avocado, chopped

**Calories:**
465

# TURKEY PESTO PASTA

For such a quick and easy meal, its popularity continues to amaze me! I think the intense flavour and speed of preparation is what makes it a hit. **Serves 2**

100 g wholewheat spaghetti
1 tbsp rapeseed oil
250 g turkey, cut in strips
50 g light cream cheese
3 tbsp sun-dried tomato pesto
1 red pepper, deseeded
  and chopped
1 green pepper, deseeded
  and chopped
1 courgette, chopped

**Calories:**
558

› Place the spaghetti in a large pot of cold water. Bring to the boil, reduce the heat and simmer until cooked.
› Place the oil in a large skillet, or pan, on a medium to high heat. Add the turkey and sauté for 4–5 minutes.
› Turn down to a medium heat and add the light cream cheese, pesto and vegetables. Sauté for a further 10–15 minutes until the turkey is cooked through and the vegetables tender.
› Once the spaghetti is cooked, drain and add to the turkey mixture.
› Serve hot.

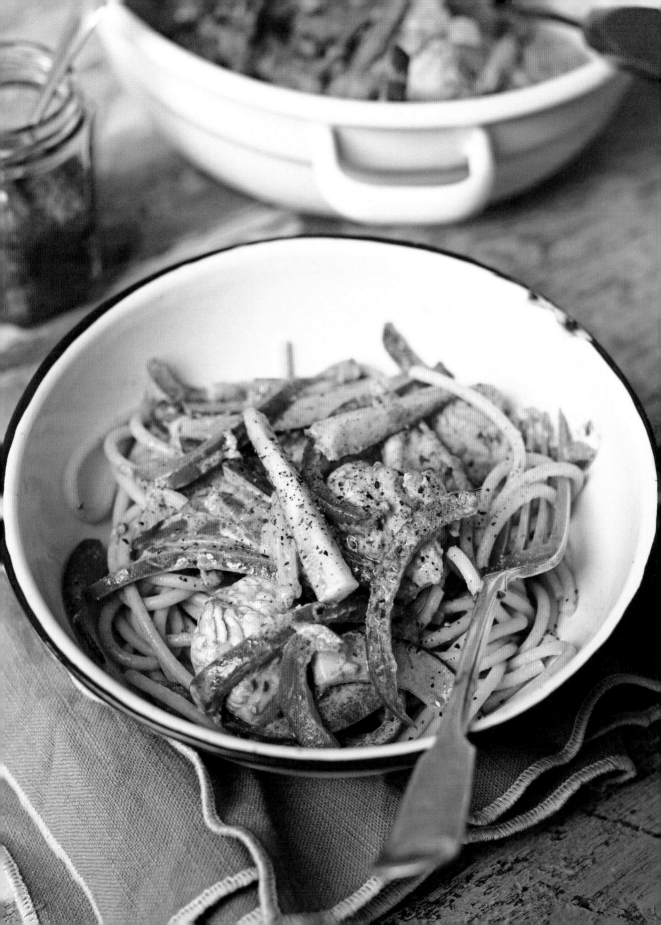

These are some great options that the little ones in the house can help to prepare and eat. Warning: it will probably get messy – but that's part of the fun, right?

# LITTLE HELPERS
# FISH GOUJONS

These homemade fish goujons can be great finger good for the younger ones in your family.

**Serves 4**

500 g fish fillets, cut in thumb-sized strips
100 g flour
pinch of salt and pepper
2 eggs, beaten
150 g breadcrumbs
2 tbsp olive oil
400 g potato, peeled
25 ml low-fat milk
10 g butter
200 g butterhead lettuce
2 tomatoes, sliced

**Calories:**
488

› Preheat the oven to 200°C/400°F/gas 6.
› Set up three bowls: the first with flour and a little salt and pepper to season, the second with the beaten eggs and the third with the breadcrumbs.
› Dip the fish strips into the flour, then the eggs and finally the breadcrumbs.
› Spread the oil over a baking tray, then lay the goujons on the tray and cook in the oven for 15–20 minutes, turning over halfway.
› Meanwhile, boil the potatoes in a pot of boiling water until soft. Drain the potatoes and then mash with the milk and butter.
› Serve with a side salad of lettuce and tomato.

# CHICKEN GOUJONS

› Preheat the oven to 200°C/400°F/gas 6.
› Set up three bowls: the first with flour and a little salt and pepper to season, the second with the beaten eggs and the third with the breadcrumbs.
› Dip the chicken strips into the flour, then the eggs and finally the breadcrumbs.
› Spread the oil over a baking tray, then lay the goujons on the tray and cook in the oven for 15–20 minutes, turning over halfway.
› Meanwhile, boil the potatoes in a pot of boiling water until tender.
› Serve with a side salad of lettuce and tomato.

Who doesn't love homemade chicken goujons? Add homemade oven chips for a treat at the weekend. **Serves 4**

450 g chicken breast, cut into thumb-sized strips
100 g flour
pinch of salt and pepper
2 eggs, beaten
150 g breadcrumbs
2 tbsp olive oil
400 g baby potatoes
200 g butterhead lettuce
2 tomatoes, sliced

**Calories:**
486

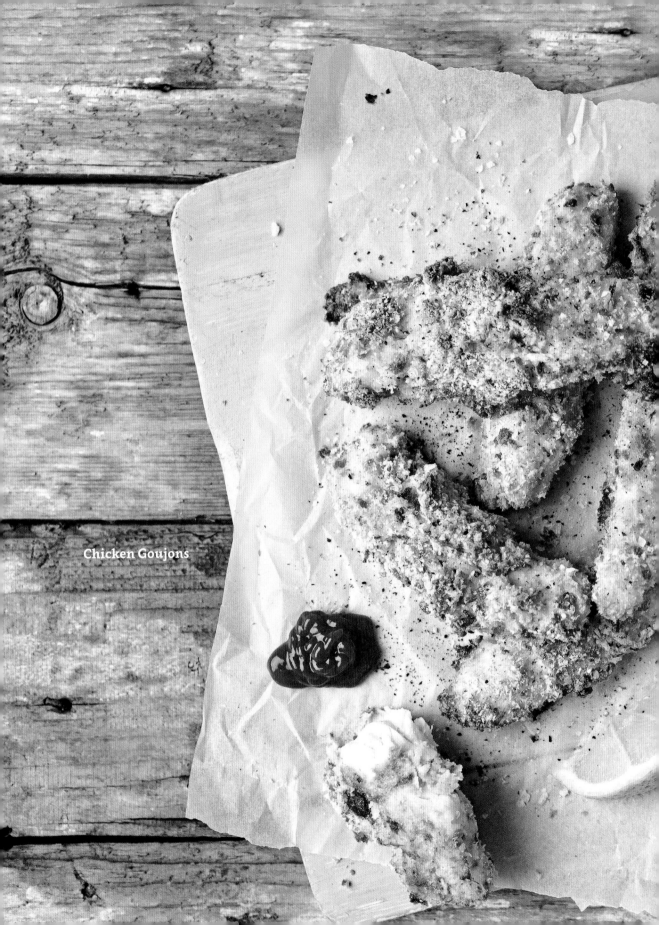

Chicken Goujons

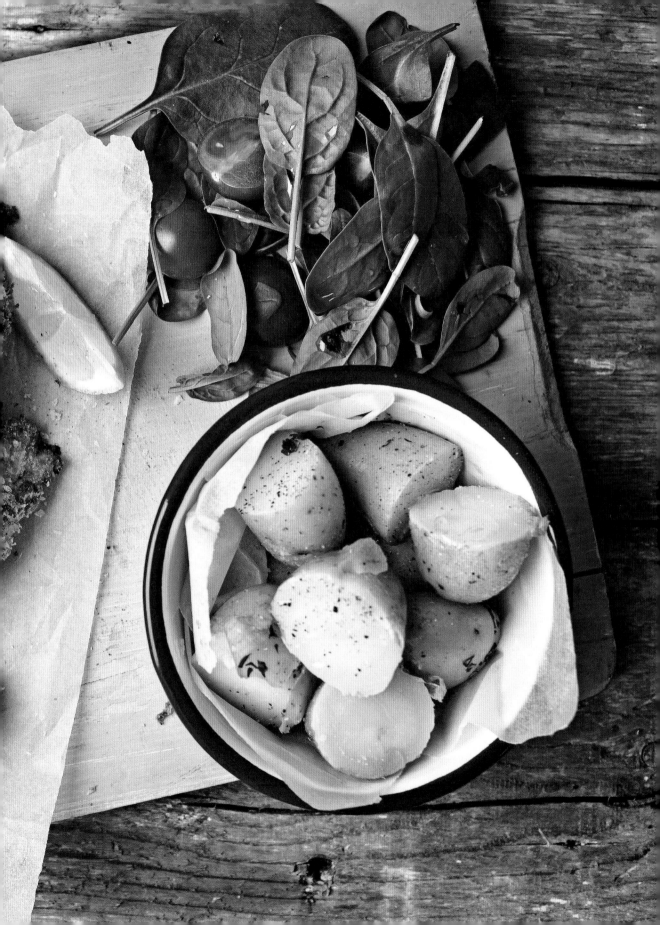

# CHICKEN KEBABS

You will need kebab sticks for this dish. Soak the kebab sticks in water for an hour – this will prevent them burning. **Serves 4**

500 g chicken breast, cut into cubes
1 red onion, roughly chopped
1 yellow pepper, deseeded and
   roughly chopped
1 green pepper, deseeded and
   roughly chopped
150 g mushrooms, halved
250 g couscous
400 ml reduced-sodium chicken
   stock, cold
60 g raisins
2 carrots, grated

**Calories:**
472

› Slide the chicken and vegetables onto the kebab sticks and grill until done on all sides.
› Meanwhile, put the couscous in a pot with the chicken stock. Bring to the boil, then turn down the heat and simmer for 20 minutes or until light and fluffy.
› Add the raisins and grated carrots to the cooked couscous.
› Serve the kebabs on the couscous mix.

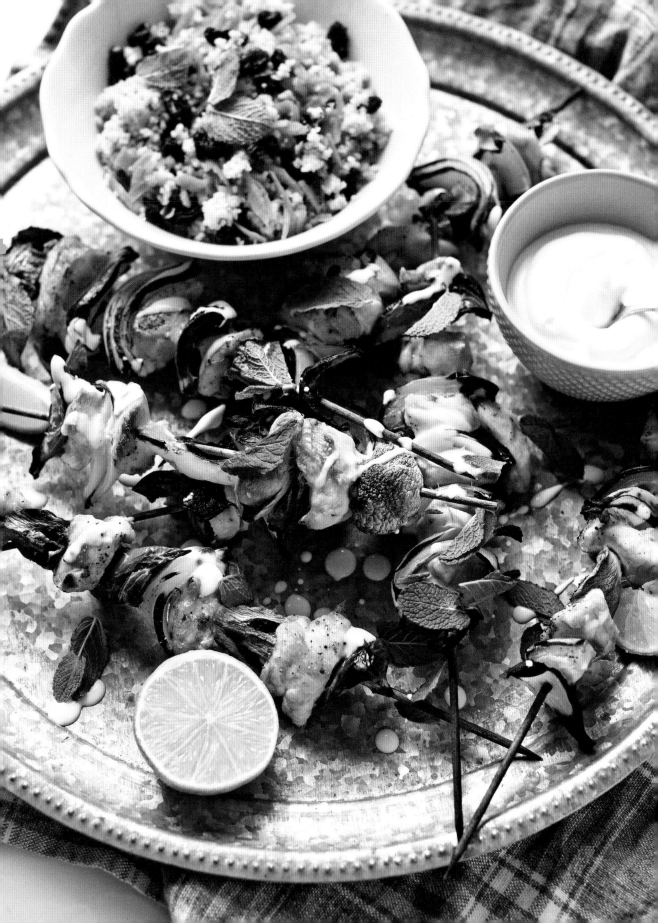

# VEGGIE PANCAKES

A great vegetarian option for the whole family. **Serves 2**

70 g flour
½ tsp salt
½ tsp pepper
½ tsp baking powder
1 egg, beaten
50 ml low-fat milk
120 g carrot, grated
120 g courgette, grated
2 onions, finely chopped
2 tbsp olive oil

**Calories:**
374

> › Mix together the flour, salt, pepper and baking powder in a bowl.
> › In a separate bowl, mix the beaten egg, milk and vegetables.
> › Then combine both bowls of ingredients together and stir until mixed well.
> › Heat half the oil in a pan and add the batter to the pan in tablespoons to make a few small pancakes at a time.
> › Cook the pancakes until golden brown on one side and then turn over to cook the other side.
> › Remove the cooked pancakes, then add the remaining oil and repeat the process until all the batter has been used.

# MEATLESS MONDAY
# PROTEIN
# SUBSTITUTES

Even if you are a meat lover like me, it is a good habit to have at least one dinner each week without meat.

If you want to substitute non-meat proteins in the preceding meals, use the options and amounts listed below. Substitutions with vegetarian protein sources can replace protein from meat sources, but they also increase the calorie content of main meals by 50–100 kcal, depending on the meal, so make sure to take that into account when calculating your meal's calorie content.

| | |
|---|---|
| Tofu (raw, firm) | 170 g |
| Tempeh | 130 g |
| Quorn mince | 210 g |
| Lentils (red, dried) | 100 g |
| Chickpeas (tinned, drained) | 200 g |

Or try out the meat-free recipes in this section.

# GOAT'S CHEESE AND BEETROOT SALAD

My unusual craving during my first two pregnancies was goat's cheese and beetroot – I couldn't get enough of the stuff. A great quick option, too! **Serves 2**

100 g wholegrain rice
50 g green salad leaves
1 red pepper, deseeded
   and chopped
150 g cucumber, sliced
150 g tomatoes, chopped
120 g goat's cheese, crumbled
100 g beetroot, sliced

**Calories:**
430

› Put the rice in a pot of boiling water and cook until light and fluffy. Once cooked, place on two plates or in a salad bowl.
› In a large bowl, combine the salad greens, pepper, cucumber and tomatoes.
› To serve, place the salad mixture on top of the rice. Then layer with the crumbled goat's cheese and beetroot.

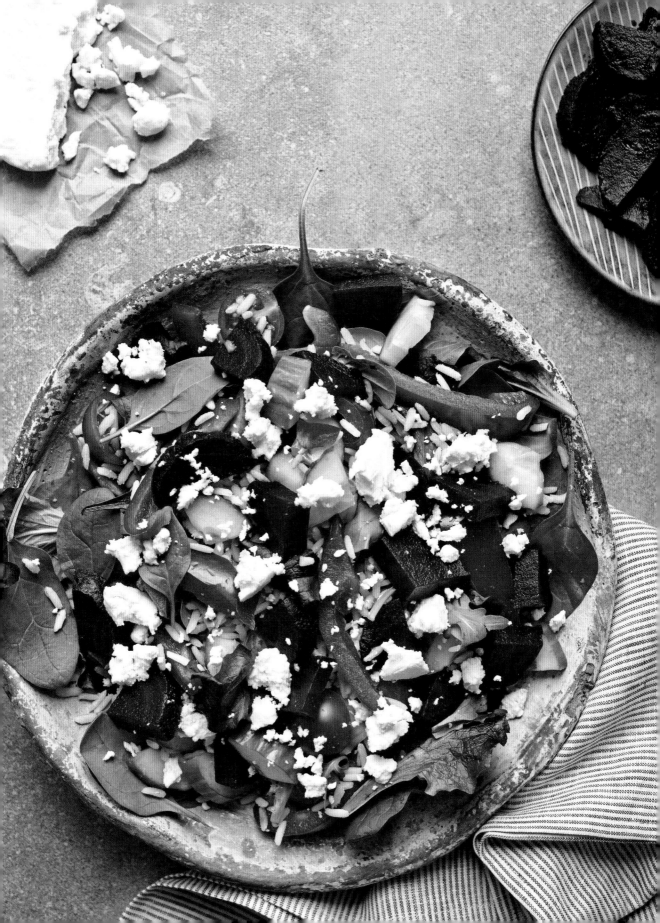

# SMOKED MOZZARELLA COUSCOUS SALAD

This recipe can double up as a great lunchtime option. **Serves 2**

100 g couscous
220 ml reduced-sodium
    vegetable stock
200 g tomatoes, chopped
1/2 cucumber, thinly sliced
1/2 red onion, finely chopped
2 sticks of celery, chopped
bunch of basil, chopped
80 g smoked mozzarella cheese,
    cubed
4 tbsp vinaigrette salad dressing
    (page 209)

**Calories:**
487

› Put the couscous in a pot with the vegetable stock, and place on a medium to high heat.
› Bring to the boil, then turn down the heat and simmer for 20 minutes, or until light and fluffy.
› In a bowl, combine all the vegetables and basil.
› Add the couscous and top with the cheese.
› Drizzle with salad dressing and serve.

# PEPPER FRITTATA

> Place the oil in a skillet, or pan, over a medium heat.
> Add the diced potato and peppers, stirring continuously for 8–10 minutes.
> In a bowl, whisk the eggs, cheese and tomatoes.
> Add the egg mixture to the pan, cooking until set.
> Once the bottom is browned you may turn it over to cook, or place under the grill (on medium heat) for 5–7 minutes, until browned on top and the inside is completely cooked and no longer runny.
> Top with the spinach and serve.

Eggs are your friend when time is tight! **Serves 2**

1 tsp rapeseed oil
200 g potato, cooked and diced
1 red pepper, deseeded and chopped
1 yellow pepper, deseeded and chopped
5 eggs
50 g Cheddar cheese, grated
2 tomatoes, chopped
50 g spinach

**Calories:**
462

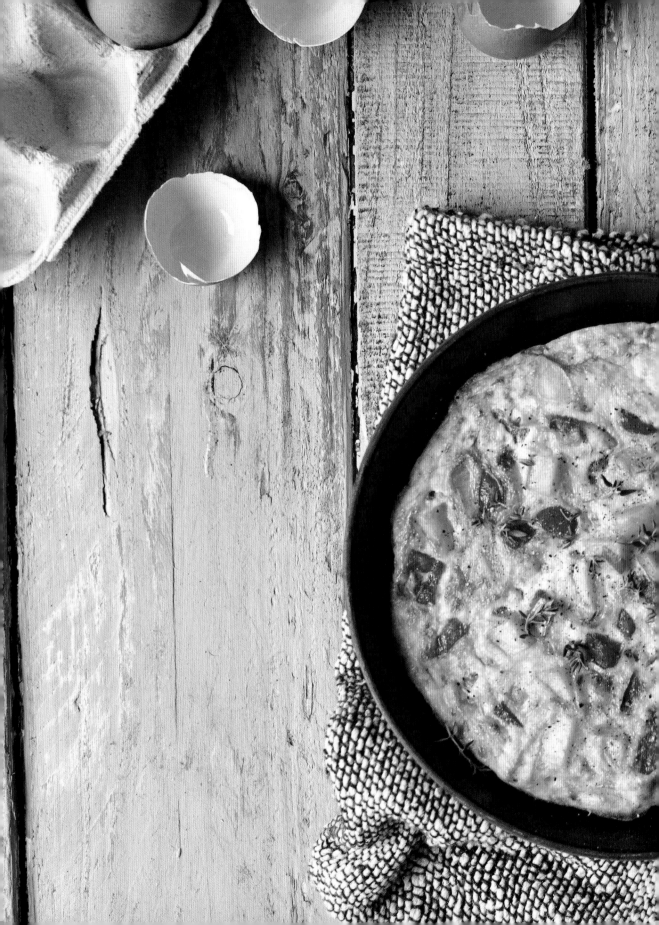

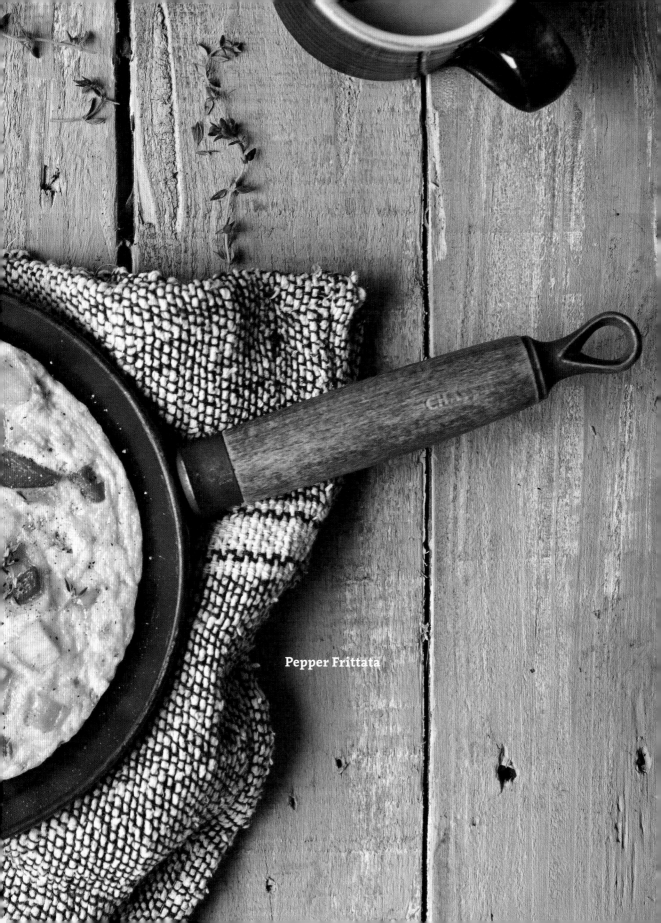

Pepper Frittata

# FALAFEL

This is a great one to make and store in your freezer for those nights when you don't feel like cooking. **Serves 2**

115 g tinned chickpeas, drained and rinsed
1/2 small red onion, chopped
1 clove of garlic, crushed
bunch of parsley, chopped
1/2 tsp cumin
1/2 tsp coriander
1/2 tsp chilli powder
1 tbsp wholemeal flour
pinch of salt
1 tbsp olive oil
2 wholemeal round pitta breads (90 g)
100 g salsa

FOR THE SIDE SALAD:
50 g spinach
100 g cherry tomatoes, halved
1/2 cucumber, thinly sliced

**Calories:**
378

› Rinse the drained chickpeas and then pat dry.
› Combine the chickpeas, onion, garlic, parsley, cumin, coriander, chilli powder, flour and salt in a blender. Blend together until smooth.
› Spoon out the mixture and form into two burger shapes.
› In a non-stick frying pan, heat the oil and then add the falafels. Fry for 3 minutes on each side or until golden brown.
› Serve with toasted pitta, salsa and salad.

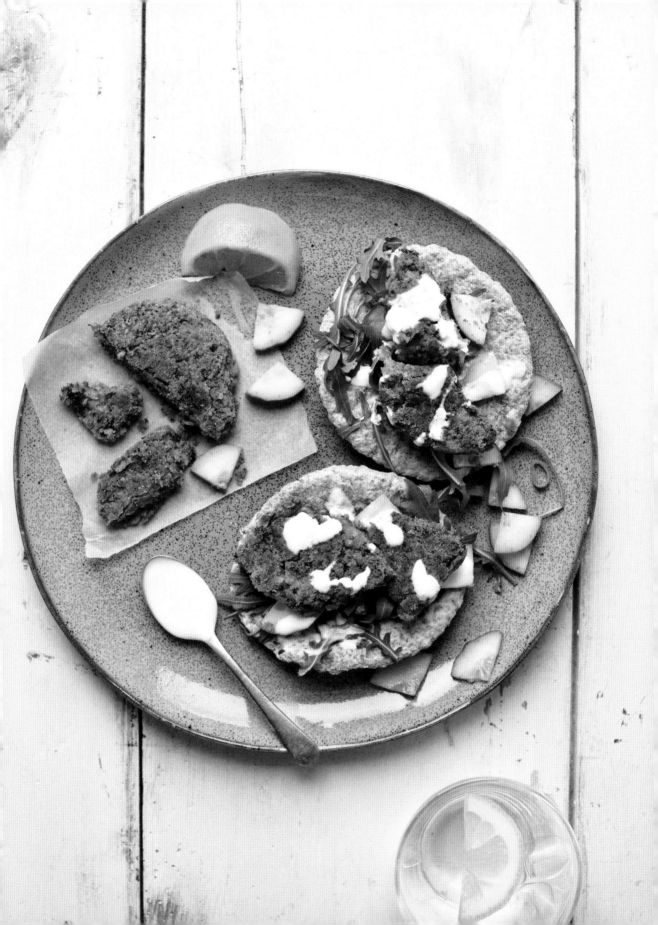

# BUTTERNUT SQUASH AND LENTIL CURRY

You can buy pre-cut butternut squash in the supermarket if you're in a rush. **Serves 2**

1 tbsp olive oil
1 small onion, chopped
$\frac{1}{2}$ butternut squash, peeled and chopped
1 tbsp curry paste
300 ml reduced-sodium vegetable stock
100 g tinned chopped tomatoes
50 g red lentils
100 g wholegrain rice
30 g natural yogurt (3% fat)

**Calories:**
492

› In a large pan, heat the oil over a medium heat. Add the onion and cook for 5 minutes, or until soft.
› Add the butternut squash to the pan and mix with the onion. Then add the curry paste, followed by the stock and tomatoes.
› Add the lentils, then bring the mixture to the boil. Reduce the heat to a simmer, cover with a lid and cook for 25 minutes.
› Meanwhile, put the rice in a pot of boiling water and cook until light and fluffy.
› Serve the rice on two plates and top with the curry. Finish with a tablespoon of natural yogurt on each dish.

# PUNCHY PASTA AND ROASTED TOMATOES

› Preheat the oven to 220°C/425°F/gas 7.
› Cut the tomatoes into quarters, scoop out the seeds and put into a sieve set over a bowl. Press on the seeds and pulp to extract the juice – you should get about ¼ of a cupful.
› Chop the tomatoes and toss with half the olive oil. Spread on a baking tray and season with a little salt and pepper. Place in the oven and bake for about 15 minutes.
› Add the pasta to a pot of water and bring to the boil, then reduce the heat and simmer until cooked.
› In another pot, heat the remaining oil over a medium heat.
› Add the garlic and cook for about 2 minutes – stir and do not allow to burn.
› When the garlic is lightly cooked, add the red pepper and courgette, and cook for 2 minutes until tender.
› Add the tomato purée and the reserved tomato juice.
› Combine the tomato sauce with the cooked pasta and roasted tomatoes.
› Serve topped with basil and Parmesan cheese.

Leftovers from this meal make an easy lunch the next day. **Serves 2**

340 g tomatoes
2 tbsp olive oil
pinch of salt and pepper
120 g wholewheat spaghetti
2 cloves of garlic, chopped
1 red pepper, deseeded
   and chopped
1 courgette, chopped
½ tbsp tomato purée
2 tbsp chopped basil
20 g Parmesan cheese, grated

## Calories:
490

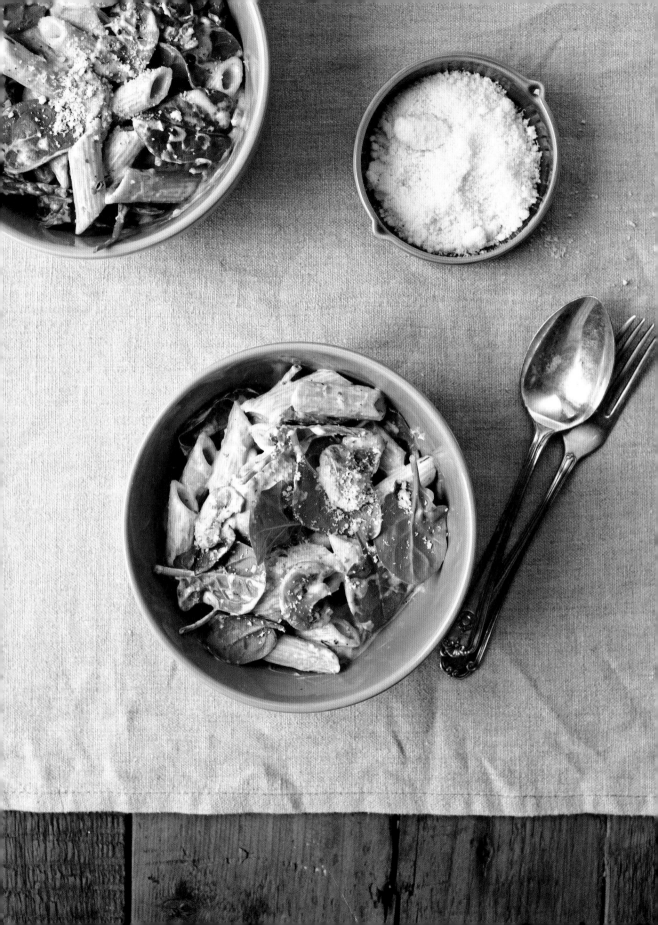

# CREAMY MUSHROOM PASTA

› Heat the oil in a frying pan on a medium heat. Add the mushrooms and cook for 8 minutes, stirring regularly.
› Then add the oregano, vegetable stock and lemon juice, and cook together for 10–15 minutes, or until the sauce has reduced by about half.
› Add the cream cheese and spinach, and cook on a low heat for 5 minutes.
› Meanwhile, add the pasta to a pot of water. Bring to the boil and simmer until cooked.
› Drain the pasta and then add it to the frying pan. Season as desired.

It's hard to believe that this is a 'healthy' meal because it is just so quick and tasty! **Serves 2**

1 tbsp olive oil
150 g mushrooms, sliced
1 tsp dried oregano
220 ml reduced-sodium vegetable stock
$\frac{1}{2}$ tbsp lemon juice
125 g light cream cheese
125 g spinach
120 g wholewheat pasta

**Calories:**
415

# COURGETTE AND CORN CHILLI

For an alternative recipe, you can make this without the chilli pepper, or to save yourself time, you can use chilli from a jar. Add hot sauce to the recipe if you like it hot!

**Serves 2**

1 red chilli pepper (optional)
200 g tinned black beans, drained and rinsed
1 tbsp olive oil
200 g sweetcorn
2 courgettes, chopped
1 onion, chopped
2 cloves of garlic, finely chopped
$1/2$ tbsp chilli powder
$1/2$ tbsp cumin
235 ml reduced-sodium vegetable stock
200 g tomatoes, chopped
1 tsp honey
bunch of coriander, chopped
juice of $1/2$ lime
pinch of salt and pepper

**Calories:**
468

› Place the chilli pepper on a baking tray and grill under a medium to high heat until it is charred all over. Remove the chilli pepper, place in a bowl, and cover with plastic until cool enough to handle. Peel and deseed the chilli pepper, then dice into small pieces.
› Place half the beans in a bowl and mash with a fork. Set aside.
› In a large pan over a medium to high heat, add the oil. Then add the sweetcorn, stirring occasionally until browned.
› After about 5 minutes, add the courgette, onion, garlic, chilli powder and cumin, stirring regularly for about 2 minutes.
› Stir in the whole beans and mashed beans.
› Add the stock, tomatoes, honey and chilli pepper, if using. Cover and simmer for 10–15 minutes.
› Stir in the coriander and lime juice.

# MOROCCAN CHICKPEA STEW

› Put the oil in a pot over a medium to high heat. Add the onion and cook until tender.
› Add the carrots and garlic, and cook for 2–5 minutes, stirring occasionally.
› Then add the cumin, crushed red pepper, chicken stock, chickpeas, tomatoes, lemon zest and potatoes.
› Simmer for 20–25 minutes until the potatoes are cooked through.
› Top with coriander and serve hot.

A hearty vegetarian stew – great for cold winter nights. **Serves 2**

1 tbsp olive oil
1 red onion, diced
200 g carrots, chopped
2 cloves of garlic, finely chopped
1 tsp cumin
$1/4$ tsp red peppercorns, crushed
470 ml reduced-sodium chicken stock
1 × 400 g tin chickpeas, drained and rinsed (240 g when drained)
200 g tinned tomatoes
1 tsp lemon zest
300 g potatoes, peeled and chopped
bunch of coriander, chopped

**Calories:**
450

Break from a traditional Saturday night takeaway and make your own! These are not necessarily the healthiest of meals but they are certainly better than ordering a takeaway. They are higher in calories than the other options, so I suggest you keep them to just once a week.

# SIZZLING STEAK FAJITAS

A Mexican-style alternative to takeaway! **Serves 2**

1 tbsp rapeseed oil
1 tbsp chilli powder
1 clove of garlic, finely sliced
300 g sirloin steak, cut into
    7.5 cm strips
1 green pepper, deseeded
    and sliced
1 red pepper, deseeded and sliced
1 onion, sliced
2 burrito-style tortillas (124 g)
30 g salsa
80 g baby spinach
2 tbsp chopped coriander

**Calories:**
590

› In a bowl, mix the oil, chilli powder and garlic.
› Place the steak, peppers and onions on a baking tray and coat with the spiced oil mixture.
› Grill on a medium to high heat until the meat is cooked through. Turn occasionally to prevent the meat and vegetables sticking.
› Serve the cooked meat on the tortillas, topped with salsa, spinach and coriander.

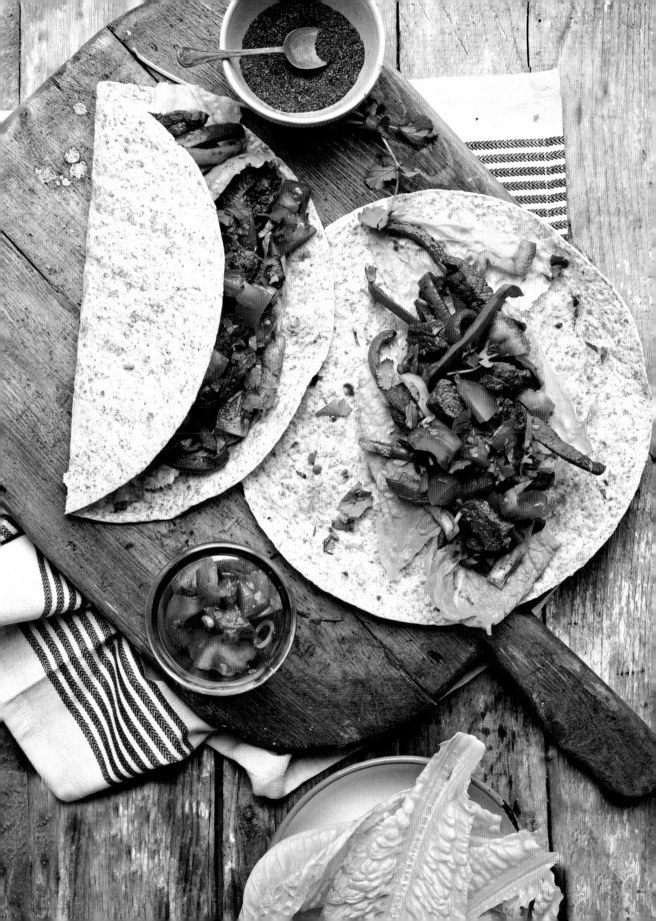

# HAWAIIAN-INSPIRED CHICKEN FINGERS AND SWEET POTATO WEDGES

Panko breadcrumbs are a Japanese style of breadcrumbs made from bread without crusts – they make these chicken fingers extra crunchy!

**Serves 2**

10 g dessicated coconut
60 g panko-style breadcrumbs
1 tsp paprika
6 tsp rapeseed oil
1 large egg
350 g chicken breast, cut into
   7.5 cm strips
200 g sweet potato, peeled

FOR THE DIPPING SAUCE:
2 tbsp sweet chilli sauce
1 tbsp mayonnaise
juice of $^1/_2$ lime

FOR THE SIDE SALAD:
50 g salad leaves
100 g cherry tomatoes, halved

**Calories:**
625

› Preheat the oven to 220°C/425°F/gas 7.
› Mix the sweet chilli sauce, mayonnaise and lime juice.
› Spread the coconut on a baking tray and place in the oven, stirring occasionally, until golden brown. Then transfer to a dish and allow to cool slightly.
› When slightly cooled, add the breadcrumbs, paprika and 3 teaspoons of oil.
› Beat the egg in a separate bowl. Dip the chicken pieces into the egg and then coat with the coconut mixture.
› Spread 1 teaspoon of oil on a baking tray. Place the coated chicken pieces on the tray and cook for 15–20 minutes, until golden brown and cooked though.
› For the sweet potato wedges, boil in a pot of water for 10–12 minutes.
› Spread 1 teaspoon of oil on a baking tray. Place the sweet potato wedges on top and drizzle over 1 teaspoon of oil. Cook for 20–30 minutes.
› Serve the chicken fingers with the salad, sweet potato wedges and dipping sauce.

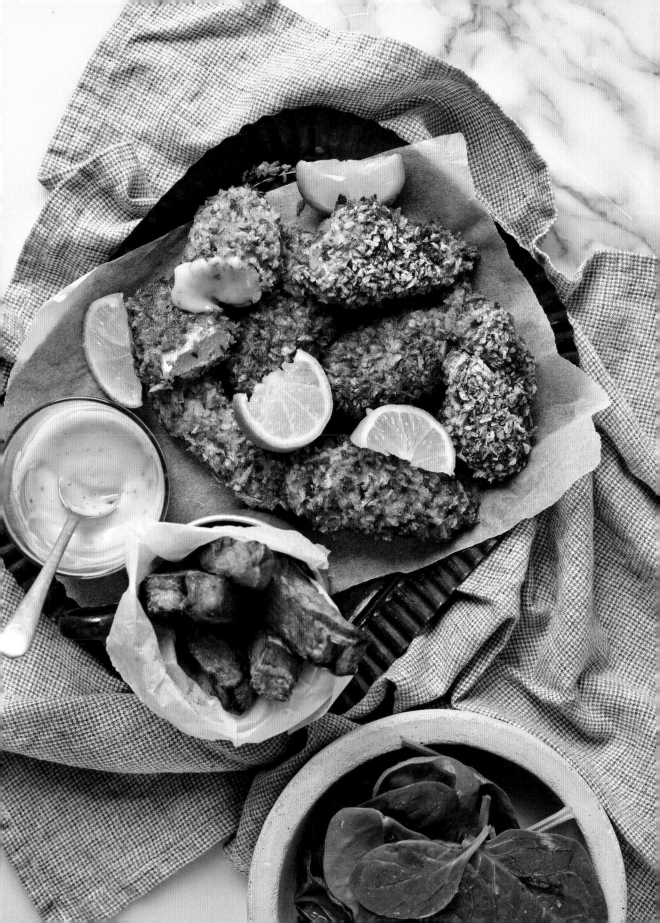

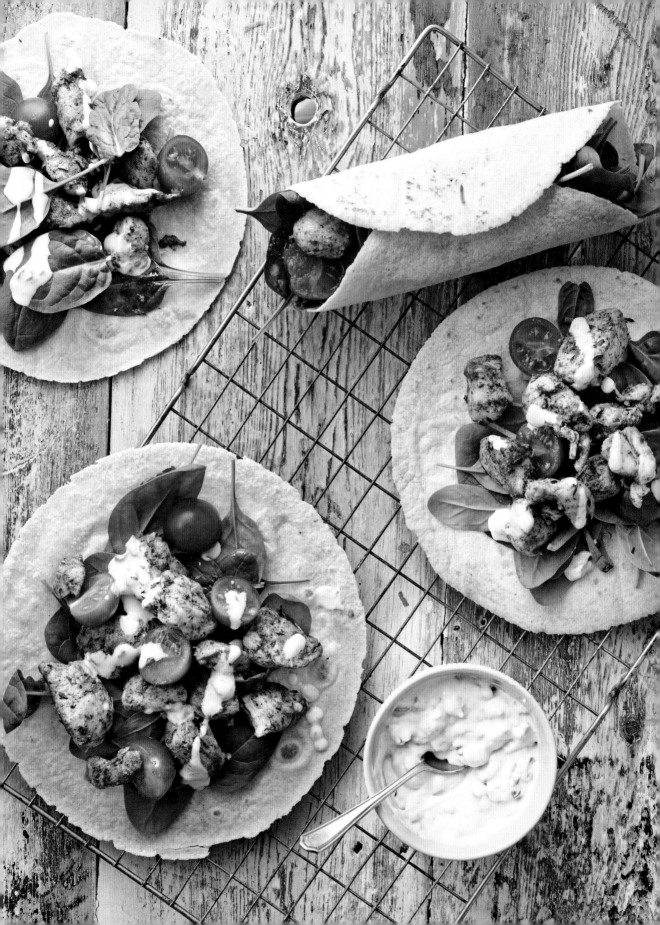

# CHICKEN TACOS

> To make the taco sauce, combine the chilli pepper, light mayonnaise, sour cream, lime juice, salt and pepper in a medium bowl. Set aside.
> In another medium bowl, combine the cumin, salt, thyme, garlic, onion, paprika, pepper, rapeseed oil and lime juice. Coat the chicken in this mixture.
> Then put the coated chicken in a pan on a medium heat and cook through.
> Fill the wraps with the chicken mixture, some of the taco sauce and coriander. Serve with the side salad.

This Mexican-inspired recipe will add a little bit of spice to your week's meals. **Serves 2**

FOR THE TACO SAUCE:
1 red chilli pepper, finely chopped
1 tbsp mayonnaise
1 tbsp sour cream
1 tsp lime juice
pinch of salt and pepper

$1\frac{1}{2}$ tsp cumin
$\frac{1}{4}$ tsp salt
$\frac{1}{2}$ tsp dried thyme
3 cloves of garlic, crushed
$\frac{1}{4}$ onion, finely chopped
$\frac{1}{4}$ tsp paprika
$\frac{1}{4}$ tsp pepper
2 tbsp rapeseed oil
1 tsp lime juice
350 g chicken breast, cut in strips
4 wholewheat wraps
bunch of coriander, chopped

FOR THE SIDE SALAD:
50 g salad leaves
50 g cherry tomatoes, halved
$\frac{1}{2}$ cucumber

**Calories:**
625

# FISH PIE

This is a great recipe for freezing uneaten portions; that way you always have a back-up, complete meal in the freezer. To increase fibre, you can make your own wholemeal breadcrumbs. Ask the fishmonger to chop the fish into small chunks to make this quicker to put together at home. **Serves 4**

300 g potatoes, peeled and
   chopped
bunch of basil, chopped, or 3 tsp
   dried basil
bunch of parsley, chopped
2 tbsp butter, softened
30 g flour
1 litre fish stock
200 ml low-fat milk
1 tbsp olive oil
600 g white fish and salmon, cut
   into small chunks
200 g green beans, chopped
1 red pepper, deseeded
   and chopped
1 yellow pepper, deseeded and
   chopped
150 g breadcrumbs

**Calories:**
623

› Preheat the oven to 170°C/325°F/gas 3.
› Boil the potatoes for 15–20 minutes until soft, then drain and mash with the basil and parsley.
› Mix the softened butter and flour together in a bowl.
› Add the fish stock and milk to a pot on a medium to high heat and bring to the boil.
› Turn down the heat to a simmer and beat in the butter and flour mixture, a small amount at a time, until the sauce thickens.
› Add 1 tablespoon of oil to a pan on a high heat. Add the fish chunks and stir gently until just cooked.
› Add the fish stock sauce and mix through. Then add the chopped vegetables and simmer for 10 minutes.
› Put the fish mixture into an ovenproof dish and layer with the mashed potato mixture.
› Top with the breadcrumbs and place in the oven for 10–15 minutes.

# THAI RED CURRY AND FRIED RICE

- › Heat 2 teaspoons of the oil in a wok, or large saucepan, for a couple of minutes.
- › Add the onion and fry for 3–5 minutes until soft and translucent.
- › Add the curry paste and cook for 1 minute, stirring all the time.
- › Follow with the chicken pieces and stir until they are coated with the paste.
- › Finally add the lemongrass, fish sauce and coconut milk.
- › Bring to the boil slowly, then reduce the heat and simmer uncovered for 15 minutes until the chicken is cooked.
- › Put the rice in a pot of water and bring to the boil. Cook until light and fluffy.
- › Add 1 teaspoon of oil to a pan over a high heat. Add the cooked rice and stir-fry for 3–4 minutes.
- › Then add the spring onions and soy sauce, and continue to stir-fry for 3 more minutes.
- › Push the rice mixture to one side of the pan, add the beaten egg to the pan and beat as if making scrambled eggs.
- › When the egg is cooked, mix it with the rice mixture, but do not mix until the egg is cooked through.
- › Make sure to stir the curry a few times while it cooks to stop it sticking.
- › Stir half the coriander into the curry and sprinkle the rest over the top. Serve on top of the rice.

So easy and tasty. **Serves 2**

3 tsp rapeseed oil
1 small onion, chopped
1 tbsp red curry paste
350 g chicken breast, cut into bite-sized pieces
1 stalk of lemongrass, thinly sliced
1 tbsp fish sauce
200 ml coconut milk
60 g wholegrain rice
2 spring onions, finely chopped
1 tsp reduced-sodium soy sauce
1 egg, beaten
2 tbsp chopped coriander

**Calories:**
635

# CHEESY NACHOS

A great dish to double the portion and share if you have guests over.

**Serves 2**

1 ¹/₂ tsp rapeseed oil
¹/₂ red onion, sliced
1 clove of garlic, crushed
1 courgette, chopped
1 chilli pepper, finely chopped
80 g sweetcorn
¹/₄ tsp cumin
1 tbsp chilli powder
200 g tinned black beans, drained and rinsed
42 g corn tortilla, cut into small triangles
30 g Cheddar cheese, grated
¹/₄ avocado, chopped
20 g goat's cheese or feta cheese, crumbled
bunch of coriander, chopped
1 medium tomato, chopped

FOR THE SIDE SALAD:
50 g baby spinach
100 g cherry tomatoes, halved
¹/₂ cucumber, thinly sliced
2 lime wedges
2 tbsp viniagrette salad dressing (page 209)

**Calories:**
640

› Place the oil in a large pan over a medium to high heat.
› Add the onion and sauté until tender. Then add the garlic and sauté for about 30 seconds.
› Follow with the courgette, sweetcorn, chilli pepper, cumin and chilli powder, and stir.
› Then add the beans and cook for 2–3 minutes until thoroughly heated.
› Cover a baking tray with tinfoil and on it place the corn tortilla wedges in a single layer.
› Grill for about 2 minutes on each side until slightly browned and crisp.
› Remove from the grill and evenly sprinkle the Cheddar cheese over the tortillas. Place back under the grill for a further 1 minute until the cheese has melted.
› Top the cheesy tortillas with the bean mixture, avocado, goat's cheese (or feta if using), coriander and tomato.
› Serve with salad and a lime wedge each.

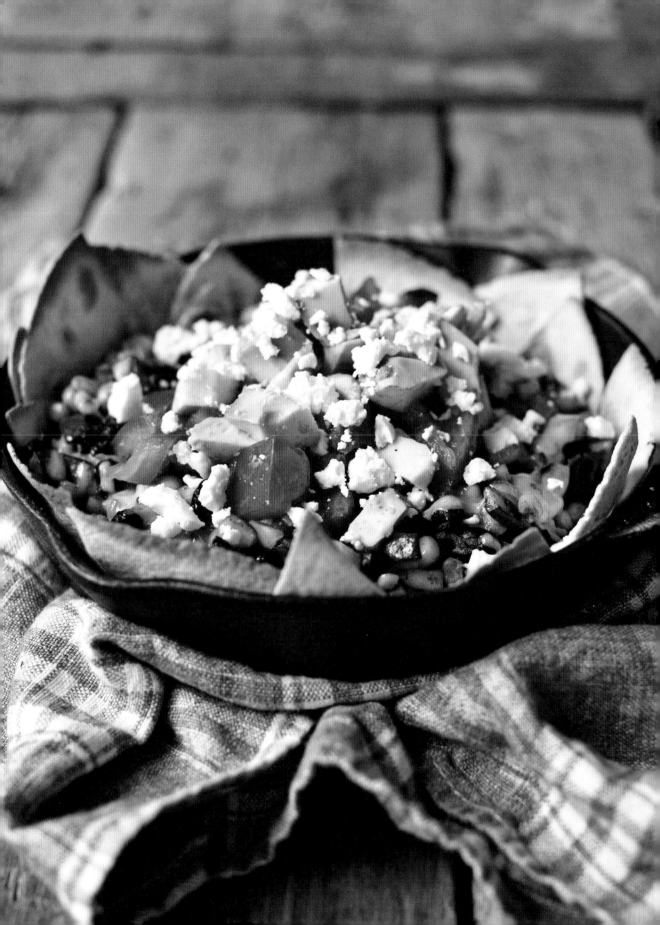

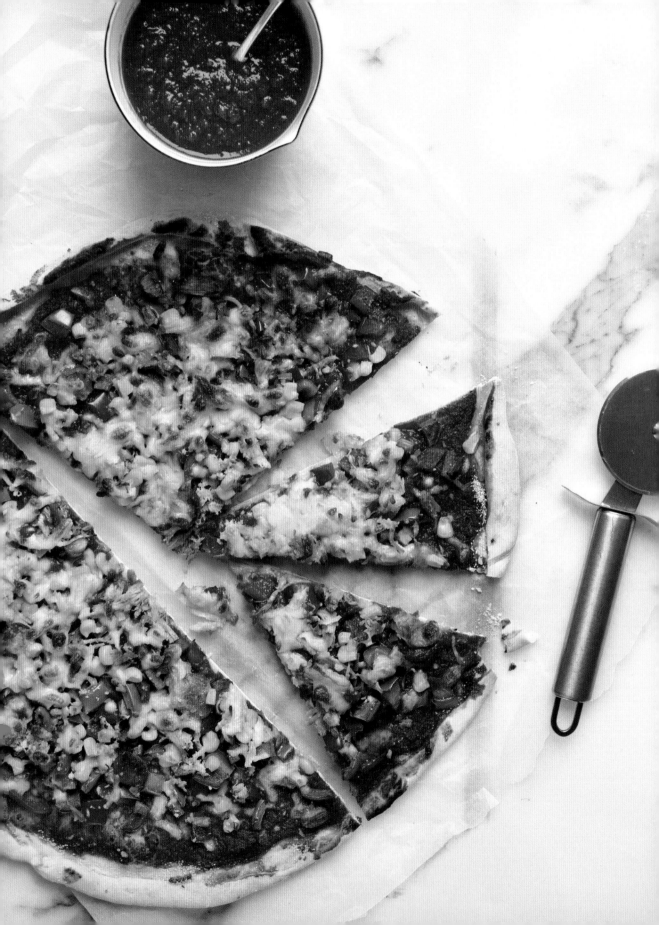

# SATURDAY NIGHT PIZZA SPECIAL

› Mix the flour, yeast and salt in a large bowl. Pour in the warm water and oil, and mix to a rough dough – it should feel damp but not overly sticky. Set aside for 5 minutes.
› Sprinkle some flour on the work surface and knead the dough for 5–10 minutes.
› Place in an oiled bowl, cover with oiled clingfilm and leave to rise until doubled in size. (You can leave it to rise in a warm room for 1 hour or overnight in the fridge.)
› Preheat the oven to 220°C/425°F/gas 7.
› Once the dough is ready, shape it into a round shape and leave for at least 15 minutes – it may take longer if the dough has been in the fridge overnight.
› Roll out into a circular shape.
› For the topping, mix the passata and tomato purée in a bowl. Spread the tomato mix on the pizza base.
› Add the rest of the toppings and then sprinkle the cheese on top.
› Place in the oven for 10–15 minutes.
› Serve with the side salad.

Leave the dough to rise overnight in the fridge, as this will boost the flavour – and it makes for quick preparation. **Serves 2**

FOR THE PIZZA BASE:
150 g strong flour
$1/2$ tsp fast-action dried yeast
$1/4$ tsp salt
100 ml boiled water, slightly cooled
1 tbsp olive oil

FOR THE TOPPING:
120 ml passata
2 tbsp tomato purée
50 g cooked ham, sliced
10 g pepperoni, sliced
1 green pepper, deseeded and sliced
1 red pepper, deseeded and sliced
1 red onion, chopped
70 g sweetcorn
sprinkling of uncooked polenta
90 g mozzarella cheese, sliced

FOR SIDE SALAD:
50 g salad leaves
50 g cherry tomatoes, halved
$1/4$ cucumber, thinly sliced

**Calories:**
620

# BEEF WITH MUSHROOM SAUCE AND SWEET POTATO WEDGES

The creamy mushroom sauce makes this dish feel more indulgent than it really is. **Serves 2**

300 g sweet potato, peeled
6 tsp rapeseed oil
pinch of salt and pepper
2 x 150 g minute steaks
400 g broccoli, chopped
100 g mushrooms, chopped
1 clove of garlic, crushed
35 g light cream cheese
30 ml low-fat milk

**Calories:**
588

› Preheat the oven to 220°C/425°F/gas 7.
› Boil the sweet potatoes in a pot of water for about 10–12 minutes. Drain the water from the sweet potatoes and chop into large wedges.
› Oil a baking tray using 1 teaspoon of the oil and place the sweet potato wedges on top. Season with a pinch of salt and pepper, then drizzle 1 teaspoon of oil over the wedges and cook for 20–30 minutes.
› Season the steak with salt and pepper.
› Steam the broccoli until tender and bright green.
› Heat 1 tablespoon of the oil in a pan on a medium to high heat. Place the steak on the pan and cook to your own liking – around 2 minutes each side for rare, 3 minutes each side for medium and 4 minutes each side for well done.
› Remove from the pan and allow to rest.
› Wipe the pan with kitchen paper and add 1 teaspoon of oil to a medium heat. Add the mushrooms and garlic, and fry for 5 minutes until golden.
› Add the cream cheese and milk. Stir until creamy.
› Serve the steaks with the sweet potato wedges, broccoli and mushroom sauce.

# CHEESEBURGER AND FRIES

› Preheat the oven to 180°C/350°F/gas 4.
› Place the potatoes in a pot of water, bring to the boil and parboil for about 10 minutes. Drain the potatoes.
› Cut the potatoes lengthways to make chips.
› Drizzle 2 teaspoons of oil on a baking tray. Put the chipped potatoes on the tray and drizzle with another teaspoon of oil.
› Place in the oven and bake for 30–45 minutes until golden.
› In a large bowl, combine the paprika, mustard powder, cumin, oregano, salt and pepper.
› Combine the minced beef, Worcestershire sauce and the spice mixture – use your hands to make sure the spices are fully mixed into the mixture. Form two burger patties.
› Put the remaining oil in a pan, on a medium to high heat, and seal the burger patties for 2 minutes on each side.
› Remove the burgers from the pan and place on a baking tray lined with tinfoil. Cover the burgers with tinfoil and bake until cooked through.
› Serve each burger on a toasted sandwich bread, topped with cheese, salad leaves and tomato. If liked, add tomato ketchup.

Yummy – need I say more? **Serves 2**

350 g potatoes, peeled
4 tsp rapeseed oil
$1/2$ tsp paprika
$1/4$ tsp mustard powder
$1/4$ tsp cumin
$1/4$ tsp dried oregano
pinch of salt and pepper
225 g minced beef
2 tsp Worcestershire sauce
2 sandwich breads (80 g)
40 g Cheddar cheese, sliced
50 g salad leaves
1 tomato, sliced
1 tbsp ketchup (optional)

**Calories:**
633

# VEGGIE BURGER

A great alternative to the traditional burger. **Serves 2**

1 × 400 g tin black beans, drained and rinsed (240 g drained)
45 g breadcrumbs
20 g onion, grated
1 tsp chilli powder (more if you like it spicy)
1 medium egg
pinch of salt and pepper
1 tbsp rapeseed oil
1 tbsp mayonnaise
dash of hot sauce
2 sandwich breads (80 g)
40 g Cheddar cheese, sliced
50 g salad leaves
85 g tomato, sliced

**Calories:**
615

› Mash the black beans in a bowl until you have a mix of mushy and whole beans.
› Mix the breadcrumbs, onion, chilli powder, egg and a pinch of salt and pepper. Add a splash of water if the mixture looks too dry. Set aside for 5 minutes.
› Divide the bean mixture into two separate balls and form two burger patties.
› Add the oil to a large pan on a medium to high heat. Cook the burgers for 4–5 minutes on each side until browned.
› In a small bowl, mix the mayonnaise and hot sauce.
› Serve each burger on a toasted sandwich bread, topped with the cheese, salad leaves, tomato and spicy mayo.

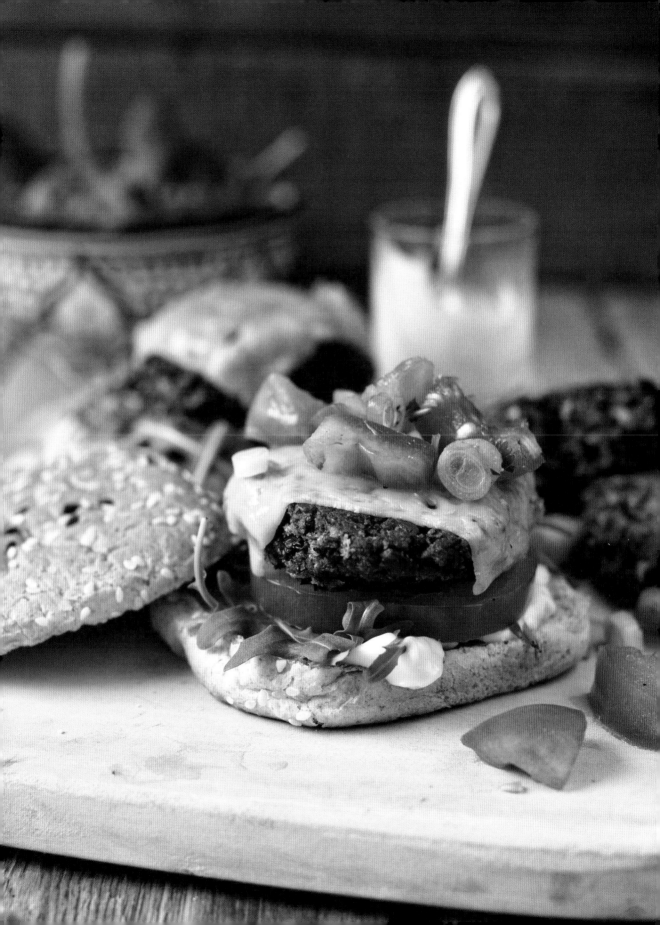

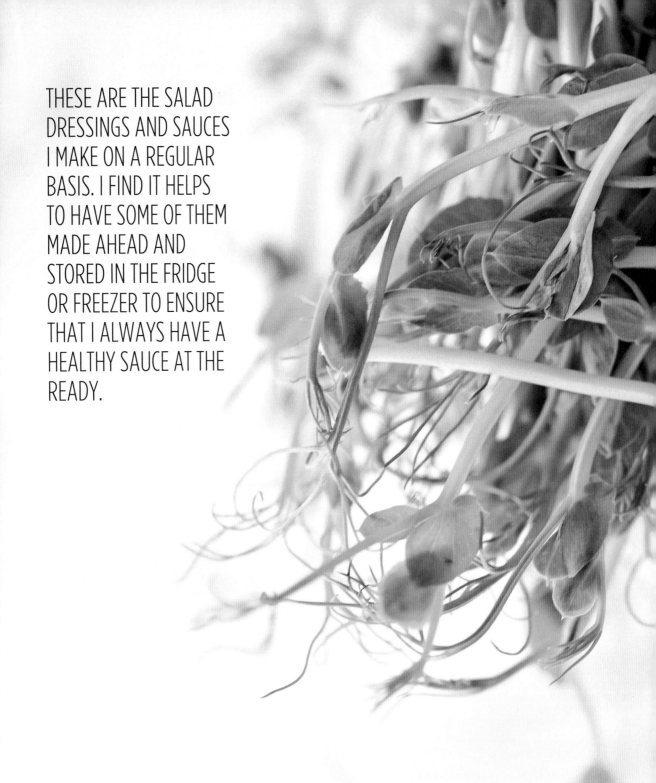

THESE ARE THE SALAD DRESSINGS AND SAUCES I MAKE ON A REGULAR BASIS. I FIND IT HELPS TO HAVE SOME OF THEM MADE AHEAD AND STORED IN THE FRIDGE OR FREEZER TO ENSURE THAT I ALWAYS HAVE A HEALTHY SAUCE AT THE READY.

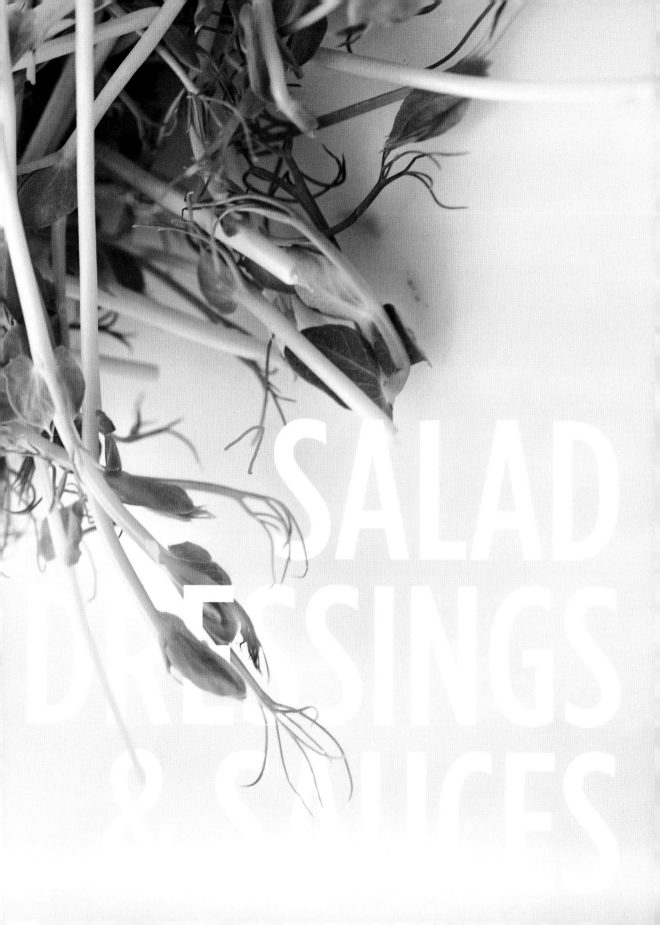

SALAD
DRESSINGS
& SAUCES

# THE BEST TOMATO-BASED SAUCE

This is my all-time favourite tomato-based sauce, which can be used for a variety of dishes. The secret to this sauce is all about the tomatoes – getting them in season is the key to the sweet, fresh taste of the sauce. Cook it slowly to let the sauce thicken naturally. **Serves 2**

1 tbsp rapeseed oil
2 cloves of garlic, crushed
$1/2$ onion, finely chopped
250 g cherry tomatoes, halved
1 tbsp tomato purée
50 g tinned chopped tomatoes
$1/4$ tsp salt
1 tsp dried basil

**Calories:**
136

› Heat the oil in a pot over a medium heat.
› Add the crushed garlic and onion, and stir over the heat until soft.
› Add the chopped cherry tomatoes, tomato purée, tinned tomatoes, salt and basil, and stir.
› Simmer on a medium heat for 5–10 minutes until the tomatoes are soft.

A tip that works really well for me is to make batches of this sauce at the time of year when you can buy local in-season tomatoes. Freeze in portions that work for you and your family and hey presto, you have a tomato-based sauce year-round!

**Mix it up:** Add some chopped chilli pepper to add an extra bit of spice, or add 35 g light cream cheese for a creamy tomato base.

# SWEET AND SOUR SAUCE

› Mix the soy sauce, vinegar, tomato purée, blended cornflour and stock.

Add extra flavour to your meat by marinating in this sauce overnight.

**Serves 2**

1 tsp reduced-sodium soy sauce
1 tbsp rice wine vinegar
1 tsp tomato purée
1 tsp cornflour, blended with water
175 ml reduced-sodium vegetable stock

**Calories:**
26

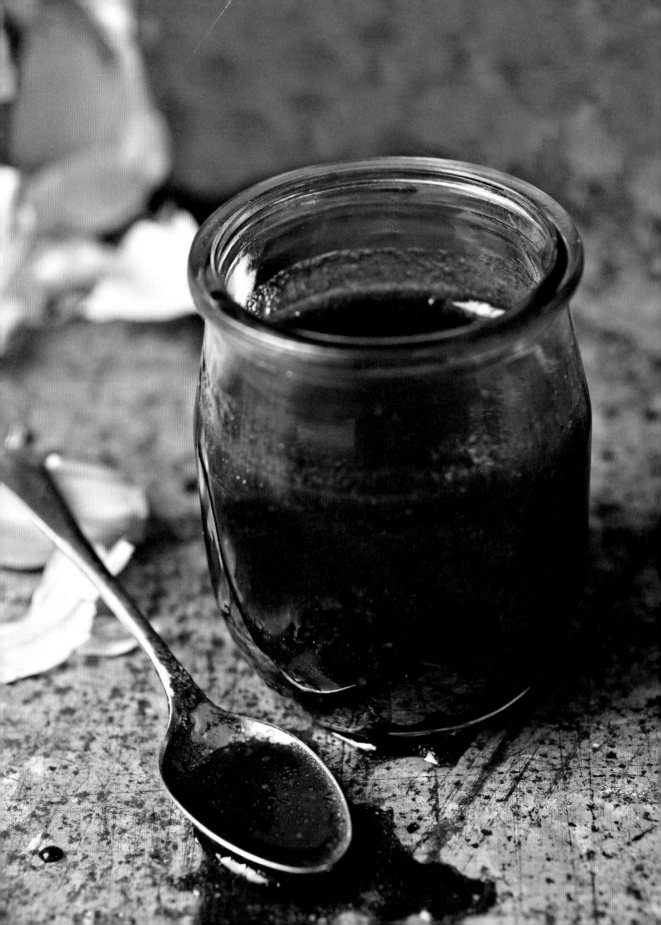

# VINAIGRETTE SALAD DRESSING

› Put all the dressing ingredients into a screw-topped jar and shake well.

I LOVE, LOVE, LOVE this dressing. I have yet to find any commercial dressing that lives up to the flavour. So even when I am tempted to take the easy option and buy a pre-made dressing, I just can't resist throwing this one together. The best bit is that as long as you have all the ingredients ready, you have it made in 2 minutes flat! **Serves 6**

50 g olive oil
2 tbsp balsamic vinegar
1 tbsp wholegrain mustard
1 tbsp honey
1 clove of garlic, crushed or
   finely chopped

**Calories:**
95

# TACO SPICE MIX

Handy to have this made in advance and stored in a Tupperware container – then you're only ever moments away from tasty tacos.
**Serves 2**

1 tbsp chilli powder
$^1/_4$ tsp garlic powder
$^1/_4$ tsp dried oregano
$^1/_2$ tsp paprika
1 tsp cumin
$^1/_2$ tsp salt
1 tsp pepper

**Calories:**
24

› Put all the ingredients in a bowl and mix well.

# FAJITA SPICE MIX

Make sure you have all these spices in your pantry so you can make this tasty spice mix in a flash. **Serves 2**

1 tsp flour
$^1/_2$ tsp chilli powder
$^1/_2$ tsp five-spice powder
1 tsp paprika
$^1/_2$ tsp cumin
$^1/_4$ tsp garlic powder

**Calories:**
21

› Put all the ingredients in a bowl and mix well.

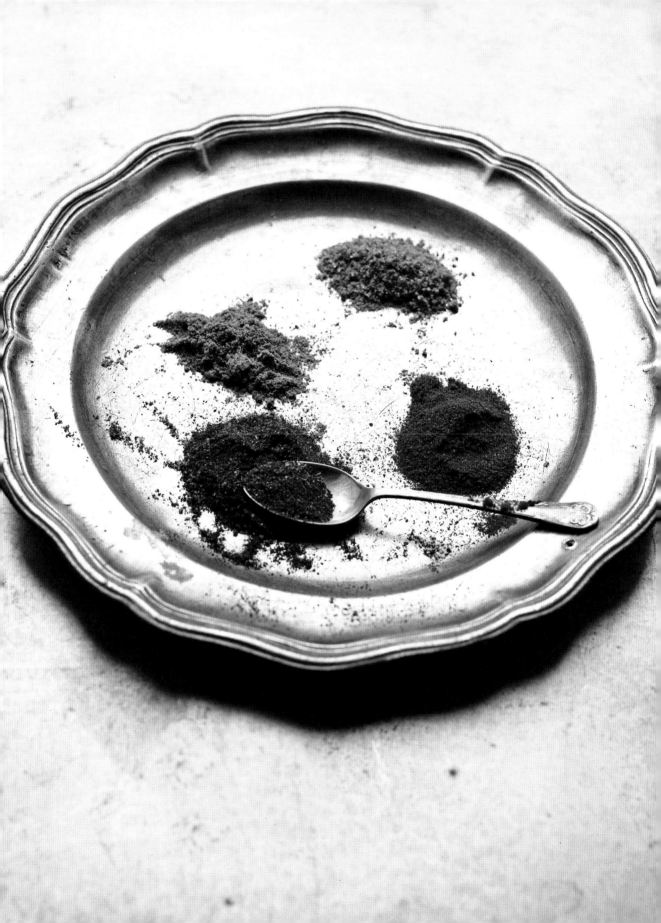

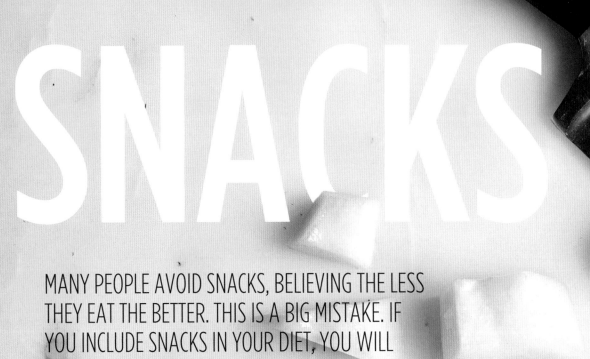

# SNACKS

MANY PEOPLE AVOID SNACKS, BELIEVING THE LESS THEY EAT THE BETTER. THIS IS A BIG MISTAKE. IF YOU INCLUDE SNACKS IN YOUR DIET, YOU WILL NOTICE THAT YOU WILL NOT NEED TO EAT AS MUCH AT MEAL-TIMES TO FEEL FULL. DON'T FORGET TO INCLUDE CARBOHYDRATE AND PROTEIN IN YOUR SNACKS, JUST LIKE YOUR OTHER MEALS. ALL SNACKS LISTED ARE AROUND 100 CALORIES AND SHOULD KEEP YOU GOING UNTIL YOUR NEXT MEAL.

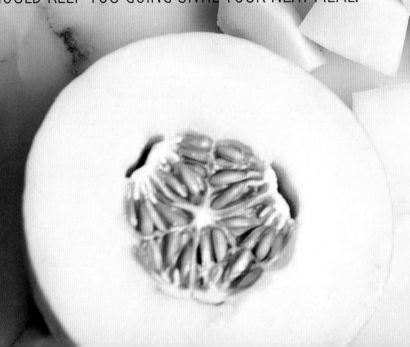

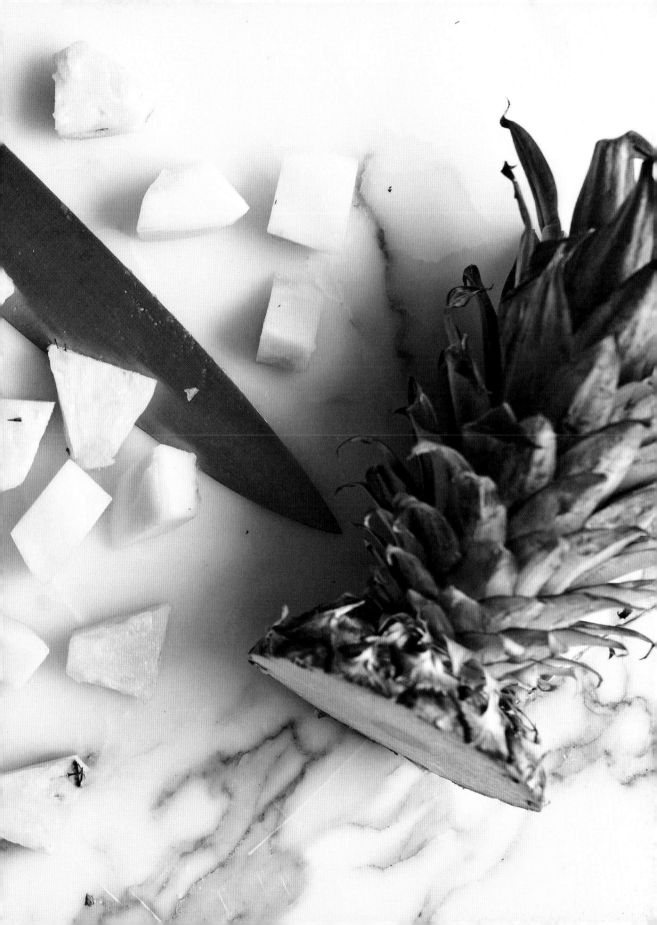

# SMOKED SALMON ROLL

A quick and easy way to get extra omega-3 fat into your day.
**Serves 1**

35 g light cream cheese
30 g smoked salmon

**Calories:**
110

› Spread the cream cheese on the salmon and roll up.

# CRACKERS AND CHEESE

By using wholewheat crackers, you will increase your daily fibre intake.
**Serves 1**

15 g cream cheese
2 wholewheat crackers

**Calories:**
116

› Evenly spread the cream cheese over the wholewheat crackers.

# FRUIT CUP

› Chop the fruit, as desired.
› Add the chopped mint leaves to the lime juice and drizzle over the chopped fruit.
› Top with the natural yogurt.

A step closer to your 5-a-day!
**Serves 1**

70 g melon
70 g grapes
4 mint leaves, chopped
juice of 1 lime
40 g natural yogurt (3% fat)

**Calories:**
90

# FRUIT AND NUTS

This is a great on-the-go snack. Remember, because nuts are a great source of good fat in the diet, they are also high in calories. It is really important to stick to the portions listed here as they all fit into the 100-calorie snack portion size. So don't guess it – measure it!

**Serves 1**

FRUIT OPTIONS (80 g):
1 apple
1 banana
1 orange

NUT OPTIONS:
6 almons
2 brazil nuts
1 tsp nut butter

**Calories:**
1 medium apple and 6 almonds 92
1 medium apple and 2 brazil nuts 125
1 medium apple and 1 tsp nut butter 122
1 small banana and 6 almonds 90
1 small banana and 1 brazil nuts 123
1 small banana and 1 tsp nut butter 121
1 medium orange and 6 almonds 101
1 medium orange and 2 brazil nuts 134
1 medium orange and 1 tsp nut butter 132

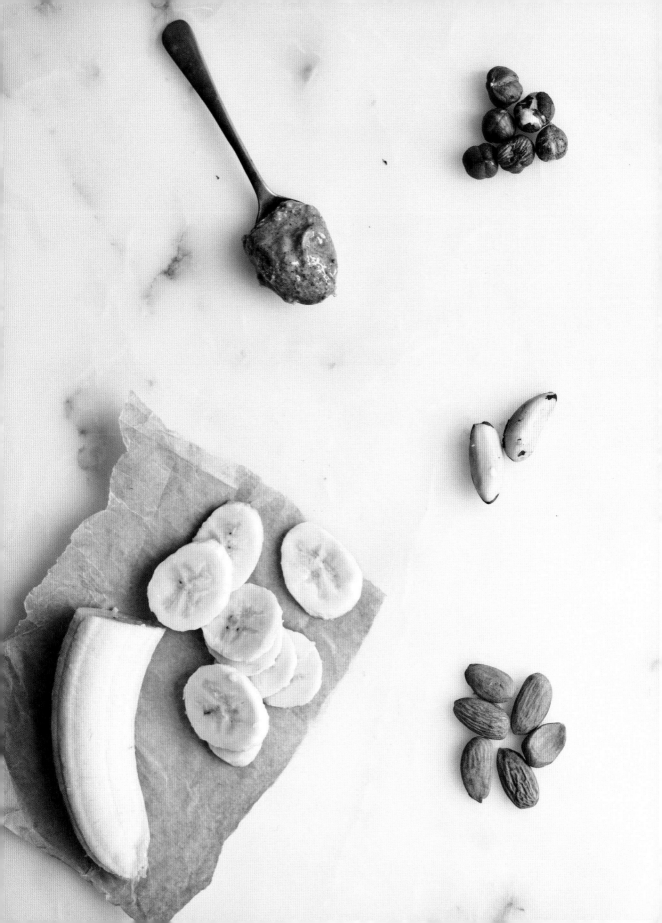

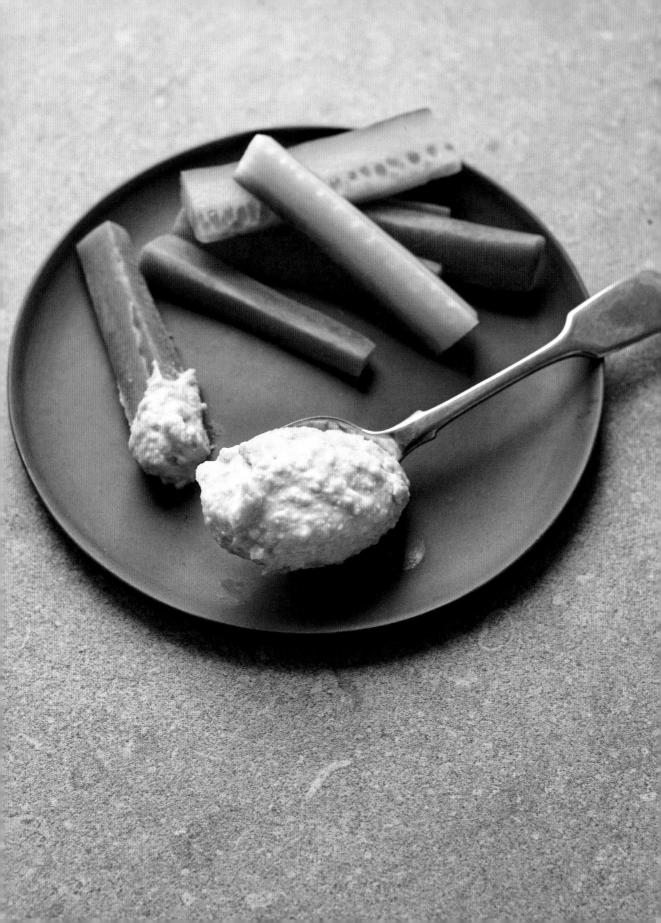

# VEGGIES AND HUMMUS

**Calories:**
1 carrot and 1 tbsp hummus 122
1 stick of celery and 1 tbsp hummus 96
1 spear of broccoli and 1 tbsp hummus 106
$^{1}/_{2}$ red pepper and 1 tbsp hummus 113

Add chilli powder or other spices to your hummus to change this one up a little. **Serves 1**

VEGGIE OPTIONS:
1 carrot
1 stick of celery
1 spear of broccoli
$^{1}/_{2}$ red pepper, deseeded and sliced

# SPINACH AND MANGO SMOOTHIE

This is one of my favourites!

**Serves 2**

60 g frozen mango, chopped
1/2 apple, cored and sliced
35 g spinach
25 g strawberries
60 g natural yogurt (3% fat)
1 1/2 tsp milled flaxseed
60 ml low-fat milk
1 tsp honey

**Calories:**
97

› Place all the ingredients in a blender and blend until completely smooth.

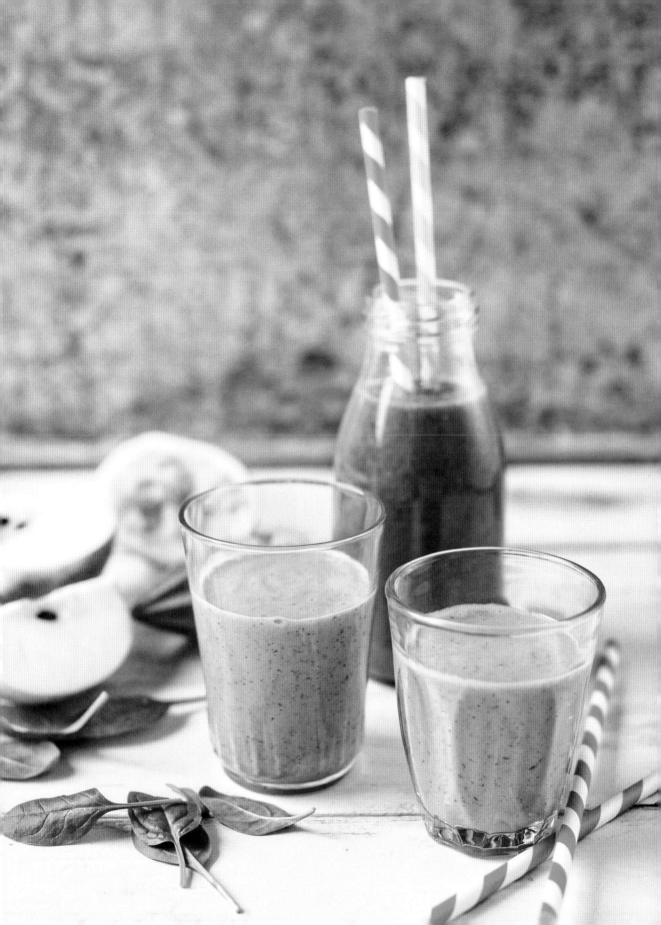

# BEETROOT AND ORANGE SMOOTHIE

A refreshing snack for hot summer days. **Serves 2**

60 g beetroot, sliced
60 ml low-fat milk
1 medium banana, chopped
1 medium orange, chopped
1 cardamom pod
7 ice cubes
$^1/_2$ tsp vanilla extract
pinch of salt
1 tbsp lemon juice

**Calories:**
117

> › Place all the ingredients in a blender and blend until completely smooth.

# BAKED BERRY SQUARES

› Preheat the oven to 175°C/350°F/gas 4.
› Mix the oats, eggs, blueberries, apple compote, brown sugar, skimmed milk, flaxseed, baking powder, cinnamon, vanilla extract and salt together in a large bowl. Then pour into a 33 × 23 × 5 cm baking tin.
› Bake in the oven until the liquid is absorbed and the oats are tender, about 25–30 minutes.
› Cut into 12 equal-sized portions.

These are a hit with everyone in my house! Another great snack that you can store in a one-serving container for a quick snack on the go. **Makes 12**

235 g rolled oats
2 eggs
90 g blueberries
120 g apple compote
40 g brown sugar
240 ml skimmed milk
15 g milled flaxseed
1 $\frac{1}{2}$ tsp baking powder
1 $\frac{1}{2}$ tsp cinnamon
1 tsp vanilla extract
$\frac{1}{4}$ tsp salt

**Calories:**
130

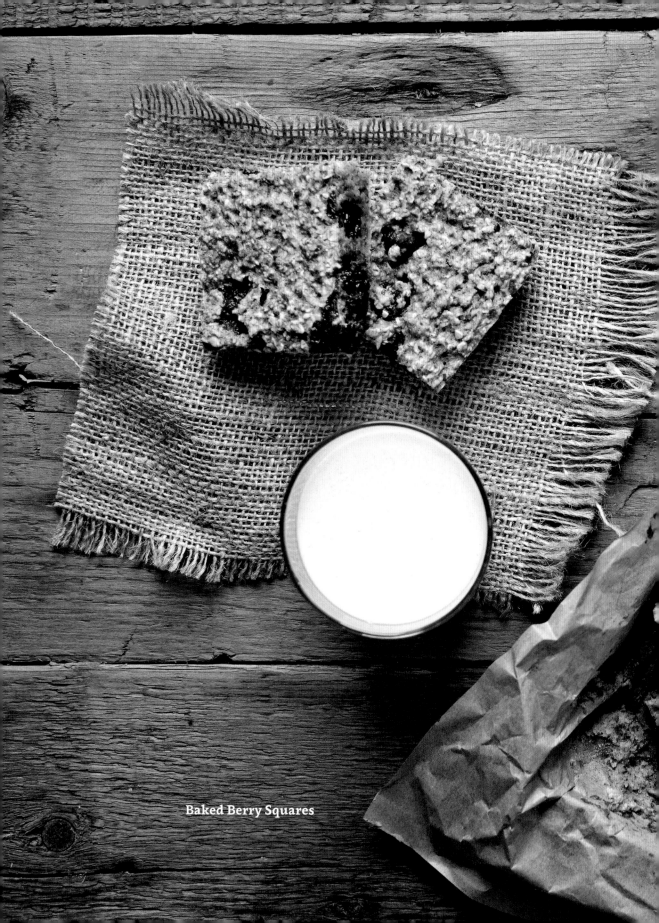

Baked Berry Squares

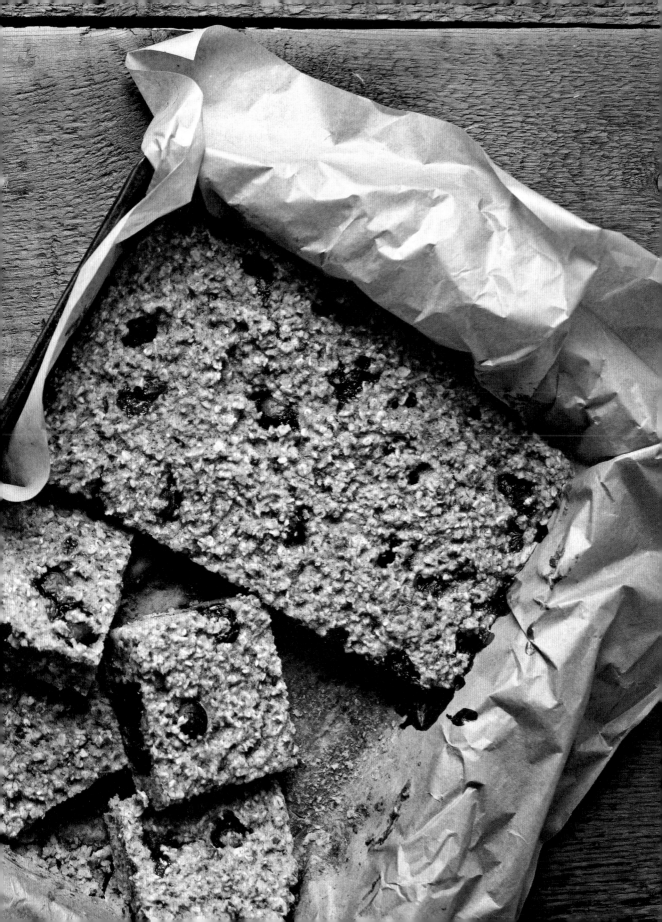

# NUTRITIONAL INFORMATION PER SERVING

Note: Sugar content reflects naturally-occurring sugar. None of the recipes contain added sugar.

## BREAKFAST

### QUICK AND EASY BREAKFASTS

| | ENERGY (kcal) | FAT (g) | SATURATED FAT (g) | CARBOHYDRATES (g) | SUGAR (g) | FIBRE (g) | PROTEIN (g) | SALT (g) |
|---|---|---|---|---|---|---|---|---|
| Porridge | 219 | 5.4 | 2.3 | 32 | 12.5 | 3.6 | 8.7 | 0.2 |
| Porridge and Banana (1 small banana) | 276 | 5.4 | 2.3 | 44.9 | 24.1 | 4.5 | 9.5 | 0.2 |
| Porridge and Strawberries (90 g strawberries) | 255 | 5.9 | 0 | 37.4 | 17.9 | 7 | 9.2 | 0.2 |
| Porridge and Raspberries (90 g raspberries) | 257 | 5.7 | 0.1 | 36 | 16.5 | 9.6 | 10 | 0.2 |
| Porridge and Blueberries (90 g blueberries) | 259 | 5.6 | 0 | 40 | 20.5 | 5 | 9.5 | 0.2 |
| Porridge and Raisins (20 g raisins) | 278 | 5.5 | 0 | 45.5 | 26 | 4.8 | 9.1 | 0.2 |
| Boiled Egg and English Muffin | 243 | 10 | 4 | 24 | 1.1 | 3.1 | 12.3 | 0.2 |
| Overnight Oats | 193 | 4.3 | 0.9 | 25 | 9.2 | 6.7 | 9.3 | 0.1 |
| Breakfast Sandwich | 217 | 6.4 | 2.1 | 26 | 3.8 | 3.6 | 11.3 | 0.6 |
| Berry and Chia Smoothie | 199 | 4.7 | 0.7 | 23 | 21 | 9.1 | 10.5 | 0.3 |

## WEEKEND BREAKFAST TREATS

| | ENERGY (kcal) | FAT (g) | SATURATED FAT (g) | CARBOHYDRATES (g) | SUGAR (g) | FIBRE (g) | PROTEIN (g) | SALT (g) |
|---|---|---|---|---|---|---|---|---|
| Hot Start | 284 | 16.9 | 5.2 | 18.4 | 5 | 4.3 | 12 | 0.6 |
| Continental Fruit Salad | 282 | 2.3 | 0.2 | 56 | 55 | 5.2 | 6.7 | 0.2 |
| Mushroom and Ricotta Omelette | 305 | 21.6 | 7.7 | 2.7 | 1.7 | 1 | 24.3 | 2.2 |
| Mixed Pepper Omelette | 344 | 20.5 | 6.9 | 13 | 12 | 5 | 23.6 | 2 |
| Goat's Cheese and Spinach Omelette | 316 | 23 | 9 | 2 | 1.5 | 1.3 | 24.2 | 1.9 |
| Bacon and Tomato Omelette | 330 | 23 | 6.5 | 5.4 | 5 | 1.6 | 24.2 | 2.8 |
| Mini Grill | 274 | 9.8 | 2.1 | 20 | 11.1 | 5 | 23 | 1.9 |
| Tropical Muesli Cup | 349 | 8.3 | 1.3 | 54 | 39 | 7.7 | 10.2 | 0.2 |
| Mediterranean Breakfast Pitta | 379 | 17.1 | 9.1 | 31 | 8.3 | 4.4 | 23 | 1.4 |
| Cinnamon and Yogurt Pancakes | 389 | 9.1 | 4.2 | 61 | 17.8 | 3.1 | 14.2 | 1 |
| French Toast | 350 | 13.5 | 5.9 | 38 | 11.1 | 6.3 | 15.4 | 1 |

# LUNCH

## SUPER SANDWICHES

| | ENERGY (kcal) | FAT (g) | SATURATED FAT (g) | CARBOHYDRATES (g) | SUGAR (g) | FIBRE (g) | PROTEIN (g) | SALT (g) |
|---|---|---|---|---|---|---|---|---|
| Base + Hot Chicken | 433 | 11 | 1 | 40 | 9 | 7 | 40 | 1 |
| Base + Chicken Salad | 395 | 10 | 2 | 34 | 4 | 6 | 40 | 1 |
| Base + Baked Ham and Cheese | 386 | 13 | 6 | 39 | 8 | 7 | 26 | 3 |
| Base + Turkey Club | 437 | 11 | 2 | 41 | 10 | 7 | 41 | 2 |
| Base + Salmon and Dill Mayo | 436 | 20 | 3 | 38 | 8 | 8 | 23 | 3 |
| Cup of Soup (200 ml of sweet potato and celery, minestrone or carrot and coriander soup) and Turkey Club Sandwich | 352 | 8.3 | 1.63 | 32 | 11 | 7 | 33 | 1.17 |
| Cup of Soup (200 ml of sweet potato and celery, minestrone or carrot and coriander soup) and Baked Ham and Cheese Sandwich | 386 | 15 | 7.53 | 34 | 12.4 | 7.3 | 25 | 3.27 |
| Cup of Soup (200 ml of sweet potato and celery, minestrone or carrot and coriander soup) and Salmon and Dill Mayo Sandwich | 304 | 11.5 | 1.83 | 30.3 | 9.1 | 6.6 | 16 | 2.27 |

## SOULFUL SOUPS

| | ENERGY (kcal) | FAT (g) | SATURATED FAT (g) | CARBOHYDRATES (g) | SUGAR (g) | FIBRE (g) | PROTEIN (g) | SALT (g) |
|---|---|---|---|---|---|---|---|---|
| Chicken Noodle Soup | 282 | 7.6 | 0.8 | 28 | 9 | 6 | 22 | 3.2 |
| Sweet Potato and Celery Soup | 186 | 4.6 | 0.7 | 30 | 11.5 | 5.3 | 3 | 0.3 |
| Butternut Squash and Vegetable Soup | 100 | 1.2 | 0.2 | 13.6 | 9.2 | 5.2 | 5.5 | 0.1 |
| Cream of Broccoli Soup | 237 | 9.6 | 2.8 | 17.1 | 4.9 | 9.6 | 14.9 | 0.9 |

| | ENERGY (kcal) | FAT (g) | SATURATED FAT (g) | CARBOHYDRATES (g) | SUGAR (g) | FIBRE (g) | PROTEIN (g) | SALT (g) |
|---|---|---|---|---|---|---|---|---|
| Minestrone Soup | 157 | 3.1 | 0.3 | 22 | 12.9 | 6.6 | 6.7 | 1.2 |
| Carrot and Coriander Soup | 136 | 4 | 2.1 | 19.7 | 11.9 | 4.4 | 2.6 | 0.2 |
| Hearty Chickpea Soup | 416 | 17.8 | 2.4 | 40 | 19.3 | 13.6 | 15.7 | 2 |
| Chicken and Lentil Soup | 351 | 3 | 0.6 | 40 | 16.4 | 6.6 | 37 | 2.9 |
| Pea and Mint Soup | 324 | 8.8 | 1.2 | 36 | 22 | 15.9 | 15.1 | 0.5 |

## SASSY SALADS

| | ENERGY (kcal) | FAT (g) | SATURATED FAT (g) | CARBOHYDRATES (g) | SUGAR (g) | FIBRE (g) | PROTEIN (g) | SALT (g) |
|---|---|---|---|---|---|---|---|---|
| Tempting Turkey Salad and Crisp Bread | 390 | 18.3 | 5.8 | 20 | 13.7 | 6.3 | 32 | 0.5 |
| Tantalising Tuna Salad | 350 | 10 | 1.6 | 37 | 18.8 | 6.4 | 25 | 0.8 |
| BBQ Chicken Salad | 380 | 10.9 | 5 | 28 | 19.4 | 8.4 | 38 | 2.8 |
| Tuna Panzanella Salad | 338 | 11.5 | 1.8 | 29 | 15.4 | 10.6 | 23 | 1.5 |
| Sunshine Salad | 200 | 7.4 | 1 | 20 | 3.9 | 5.1 | 9.5 | 0.1 |
| Caprese Pasta Salad | 395 | 23 | 7.7 | 29 | 10.7 | 4.4 | 16.3 | 1.4 |
| Tomato and Avocado Salad | 370 | 32 | 5.3 | 12.1 | 10.6 | 6.1 | 3.9 | 2.7 |
| Spinach Salad with Chicken, Corn and Feta | 398 | 12.9 | 3.8 | 32 | 17.7 | 9.8 | 33 | 1.6 |
| Baked Tomatoes with Goat's Cheese | 388 | 18.5 | 7 | 36 | 16 | 7.5 | 13.6 | 1 |
| Cajun-Grilled Chicken and Black-Eyed Bean Salad | 445 | 10 | 1.7 | 39 | 6.3 | 12.4 | 43 | 2.1 |

# DINNER

BEEF

| | ENERGY (kcal) | FAT (g) | SATURATED FAT (g) | CARBOHYDRATES (g) | SUGAR (g) | FIBRE (g) | PROTEIN (g) | SALT (g) |
|---|---|---|---|---|---|---|---|---|
| Lasagne and Salad | 554 | 21 | 8.2 | 49 | 23 | 11.3 | 35 | 0.8 |
| Curry Beef Noodle Bowl | 530 | 20 | 3 | 46 | 7.9 | 8.4 | 35 | 2.9 |
| Spaghetti Bolognese | 451 | 10.5 | 3.1 | 49 | 17.7 | 13 | 33 | 0.8 |
| Ginger Beef | 509 | 14 | 3.3 | 49 | 11.4 | 10.7 | 40 | 0.2 |
| Cottage Pie | 517 | 26 | 12.7 | 38 | 13.9 | 6.8 | 28 | 1.3 |
| Beef and Rice | 545 | 18.7 | 6 | 52 | 19.8 | 8.5 | 38 | 0.9 |
| Italian Steak | 428 | 13.4 | 3.2 | 32 | 8.4 | 11.3 | 38 | 0.7 |
| Meatballs and Spaghetti | 552 | 16.9 | 4.5 | 52 | 17.7 | 13 | 40 | 0.9 |
| Pot Roast | 424 | 12.2 | 3.4 | 36 | 14.9 | 7 | 38 | 0.3 |
| Chilli | 471 | 17.1 | 6.3 | 34 | 11 | 10.2 | 39 | 2 |
| Beef Lo Mein | 502 | 10.5 | 2.8 | 56 | 13.6 | 18.9 | 35 | 1.9 |
| Buffalo Steak and Corn | 467 | 20 | 8.7 | 33 | 2.2 | 5.4 | 35 | 1.4 |

| | ENERGY (kcal) | FAT (g) | SATURATED FAT (g) | CARBOHYDRATES (g) | SUGAR (g) | FIBRE (g) | PROTEIN (g) | SALT (g) |
|---|---|---|---|---|---|---|---|---|
| Sea Bass with Salsa-Inspired Sauce | 557 | 17 | 2.2 | 61 | 15.7 | 7 | 35 | 32 |
| Mexican Cod | 526 | 18.2 | 1.7 | 43 | 14.9 | 13.3 | 39 | 3.3 |
| Sun-Dried Tomato Salmon | 540 | 27 | 4.6 | 29 | 5.1 | 10.6 | 37 | 0.5 |
| Salmon and Couscous | 512 | 26 | 4.1 | 32 | 10.6 | 8.3 | 32 | 0.8 |
| Quick Fish Stew | 533 | 14.1 | 2.5 | 51 | 14.8 | 8 | 46 | 1.6 |
| Quick Tuna Pasta | 496 | 14.8 | 8.2 | 52 | 16.3 | 11.6 | 32 | 3 |
| Seafood Curry | 557 | 10.3 | 1 | 73 | 13 | 8.4 | 38 | 1.2 |
| Mackerel and Quinoa | 530 | 30 | 6 | 28 | 8.7 | 5.7 | 34 | 0.8 |
| Haddock with Coconut Rice | 426 | 12.4 | 1.6 | 42 | 5.9 | 4.1 | 35 | 0.5 |
| Teriyaki Salmon and Coriander Rice | 549 | 21 | 3.9 | 48 | 17.6 | 7.1 | 37 | 2.6 |
| Chilli Salmon Noodle Bowl | 495 | 14 | 2.6 | 53 | 14.4 | 6 | 36 | 4.1 |
| Indian Fish Curry | 539 | 22 | 12.8 | 46 | 21 | 9.7 | 34 | 1 |
| Fish Cakes and Salad | 510 | 14.9 | 2.1 | 54 | 13.4 | 7.3 | 36 | 1.8 |
| Curry Coconut Fish Parcel | 505 | 7.1 | 1.9 | 64 | 21 | 11 | 39 | 1.2 |

## PORK

|  | ENERGY (kcal) | FAT (g) | SATURATED FAT (g) | CARBOHYDRATES (g) | SUGAR (g) | FIBRE (g) | PROTEIN (g) | SALT (g) |
|---|---|---|---|---|---|---|---|---|
| Pork Tenderloin with Orange Marinade | 404 | 6.1 | 1.7 | 48 | 21 | 7.1 | 35 | 4.4 |
| Spicy Pork and Carrot Stir-Fry | 554 | 14.7 | 3.1 | 50 | 13 | 8 | 51 | 1.7 |
| Sweet and Sour Pork | 510 | 13.2 | 2.6 | 51 | 10.7 | 8 | 42 | 1.4 |
| Pork Medallions with Super Green Sauce | 436 | 12.9 | 3.1 | 35 | 12.4 | 6.6 | 41 | 2 |
| Pork with Sprouts | 511 | 13.5 | 3 | 46 | 9.1 | 9.1 | 46 | 3.4 |
| Pork Steak with Peppers and Creamy Polenta | 367 | 10.2 | 3.2 | 32 | 10.6 | 3.6 | 35 | 0.7 |

## POULTRY

|  | ENERGY (kcal) | FAT (g) | SATURATED FAT (g) | CARBOHYDRATES (g) | SUGAR (g) | FIBRE (g) | PROTEIN (g) | SALT (g) |
|---|---|---|---|---|---|---|---|---|
| Chicken and Chorizo Pasta Bake | 551 | 26 | 5.6 | 36 | 13.6 | 11.3 | 37 | 2.2 |
| Herby Roast Chicken | 403 | 11.9 | 3.6 | 47 | 20 | 11.6 | 19.7 | 0.3 |
| Chicken and Loaded-Vegetable Bake | 543 | 14 | 7.4 | 51 | 17.6 | 14 | 44 | 0.8 |
| Mango Chicken | 548 | 12.5 | 1.4 | 60 | 2 | 10.3 | 42 | 2.5 |
| Chicken and Ginger Curry | 553 | 14.5 | 1.4 | 54 | 20 | 9.9 | 46 | 1.5 |
| Chicken Fajitas | 532 | 13.3 | 2.6 | 53 | 22 | 10.9 | 43 | 2.6 |
| Chicken Quesadillas and Salad | 530 | 15.2 | 2.9 | 53 | 24 | 12.5 | 44 | 1.7 |
| Spanish Chicken | 547 | 10.4 | 1.2 | 65 | 24 | 12.6 | 41 | 1.1 |
| Stuffed Chicken with Lemon, Capers and Chilli | 452 | 15.6 | 3.7 | 30 | 10.7 | 8.3 | 43 | 0.6 |
| Granny Brid's Chicken | 492 | 17.3 | 5 | 32 | 8 | 4 | 50 | 0.5 |
| Tex Mex Chicken and Wholewheat Noodles | 509 | 9.1 | 1.8 | 55 | 16.8 | 8.6 | 46 | 1.4 |

| | ENERGY (kcal) | FAT (g) | SATURATED FAT (g) | CARBOHYDRATES (g) | SUGAR (g) | FIBRE (g) | PROTEIN (g) | SALT (g) |
|---|---|---|---|---|---|---|---|---|
| Roast Basil Chicken | 439 | 11 | 4.1 | 18.3 | 6.4 | 4.2 | 64 | 0.5 |
| Five-Spice Chicken | 476 | 11.4 | 2 | 36 | 3 | 6 | 54 | 2.8 |
| Roast Italian-Style Spicy Chicken | 480 | 11 | 2.4 | 27 | 9.5 | 4.7 | 65 | 0.4 |
| Spanish Chicken Stew with Chickpeas | 412 | 13.8 | 3.8 | 30 | 16.1 | 9 | 36 | 1.5 |
| Chicken Parmesan | 505 | 14.2 | 4.1 | 36 | 7 | 6.8 | 54 | 1 |
| Grilled Chicken and Sweetcorn Salad with Chilli Cream Dressing | 465 | 28 | 7.5 | 20 | 10.4 | 6 | 29 | 1.6 |
| Turkey Pesto Pasta | 558 | 21 | 4.3 | 41 | 11.5 | 12.3 | 43 | 0.8 |

## LITTLE HELPERS

| | ENERGY (kcal) | FAT (g) | SATURATED FAT (g) | CARBOHYDRATES (g) | SUGAR (g) | FIBRE (g) | PROTEIN (g) | SALT (g) |
|---|---|---|---|---|---|---|---|---|
| Fish Goujons | 488 | 13 | 3 | 56 | 5 | 4.5 | 33 | 0.9 |
| Chicken Goujons | 486 | 11.3 | 2.1 | 54 | 6.1 | 5.3 | 38 | 1 |
| Chicken Kebabs | 472 | 3.7 | 0.8 | 65 | 19.8 | 7.4 | 41 | 0.5 |
| Veggie Pancakes | 374 | 16.8 | 3 | 39 | 17.8 | 9.7 | 11 | 2.7 |

## MEATLESS MONDAY

| | ENERGY (KCAL) | FAT (G) | SATURATED FAT (G) | CARBOHYDRATES (G) | SUGAR (G) | FIBRE (G) | PROTEIN (G) | SALT (G) |
|---|---|---|---|---|---|---|---|---|
| Goat's Cheese and Beetroot Salad | 430 | 16.8 | 11 | 47 | 11.6 | 6.3 | 19.4 | 1 |
| Smoked Mozzarella Couscous Salad | 487 | 23 | 7.6 | 48 | 14 | 7.6 | 16.9 | 1.76 |
| Pepper Frittata | 462 | 24 | 9.3 | 29 | 11.5 | 7 | 28 | 1 |
| Falafel | 378 | 9.8 | 1.4 | 54 | 9.8 | 10.3 | 12.9 | 3.1 |
| Butternut Squash and Lentil Curry | 492 | 12.5 | 1.1 | 75 | 17 | ;4 | 16 | 0.9 |
| Punchy Pasta and Roasted Tomatoes | 490 | 21 | 4.4 | 52 | 15.7 | 12.9 | 16 | 0.3 |
| Creamy Mushroom Pasta | 415 | 16.9 | 6 | 43 | 6.5 | 10.2 | 16.8 | 0.9 |
| Courgette and Corn Chilli | 468 | 9.7 | 1.5 | 65 | 24 | 19.8 | 18 | 2.2 |
| Moroccan Chickpea Stew | 450 | 12.6 | 1.9 | 58 | 15 | 12 | 19.7 | 1.8 |

## SATURDAY TAKEWAY MEALS

| | ENERGY (kcal) | FAT (g) | SATURATED FAT (g) | CARBOHYDRATES (g) | SUGAR (g) | FIBRE (g) | PROTEIN (g) | SALT (g) |
|---|---|---|---|---|---|---|---|---|
| Sizzling Steak Fajitas | 590 | 21 | 5.2 | 49 | 16.7 | 10.4 | 45 | 2.5 |
| Hawaiian-Inspired Chicken Fingers and Sweet Potato Wedges | 625 | 22 | 5.1 | 53 | 17.9 | 5.4 | 51 | 0.9 |
| Chicken Tacos | 625 | 32 | 5.9 | 41 | 6.5 | 6.5 | 39 | 2 |
| Fish Pie | 623 | 24 | 7.3 | 55 | 11.8 | 7.4 | 42 | 2.6 |
| Thai Red Curry and Fried Rice | 635 | 34 | 17.7 | 30 | 4.7 | 2 | 51 | 3.3 |
| Cheesy Nachos | 640 | 26 | 7.8 | 66 | 17.2 | 18 | 24 | 2.5 |
| Saturday Night Pizza Special | 620 | 17.2 | 5.7 | 81 | 23 | 8.7 | 30 | 2.2 |
| Beef with Mushroom Sauce and Sweet Potato Wedges | 588 | 25 | 6.4 | 37 | 13.5 | 11.8 | 46 | 1.1 |
| Cheeseburger and Fries | 633 | 28 | 9.9 | 53 | 7.9 | 6.2 | 39 | 1.8 |
| Veggie Burger | 615 | 25 | 6.4 | 64 | 4.5 | 14.4 | 26 | 2.1 |

# SALAD DRESSINGS AND SAUCES

| | ENERGY (kcal) | FAT (g) | SATURATED FAT (g) | CARBOHYDRATES (g) | SUGAR (g) | FIBRE (g) | PROTEIN (g) | SALT (g) |
|---|---|---|---|---|---|---|---|---|
| The Best Tomato-Based Sauce | 136 | 7.2 | 0.5 | 11.9 | 10.9 | 3.9 | 3.5 | 0.5 |
| Sweet and Sour Sauce | 26 | 0.2 | 0 | 4.6 | 2.8 | 1.1 | 0.9 | 1 |
| Vinaigrette Salad Dressing | 95 | 8.7 | 1.2 | 3.7 | 3.5 | 0 | 0.5 | 0.2 |
| Taco Spice Mix | 24 | 1.2 | 0.2 | 0.6 | 0.4 | 2.3 | 1.3 | 1.7 |
| Fajita Spice Mix | 21 | 0.5 | 0.1 | 3 | 0.2 | 0.8 | 0.8 | 0.1 |

# SNACKS

| | ENERGY (kcal) | FAT (g) | SATURATED FAT (g) | CARBOHYDRATES (g) | SUGAR (g) | FIBRE (g) | PROTEIN (g) | SALT (g) |
|---|---|---|---|---|---|---|---|---|
| Smoked Salmon Roll | 110 | 5.5 | 2.2 | 2.8 | 2.6 | 0 | 12.1 | 1.5 |
| Crackers and Cheese | 116 | 6.1 | 3.8 | 8.8 | 2.4 | 0.7 | 6.1 | 0.5 |
| Fruit Cup | 90 | 0.3 | 0 | 17.9 | 17.6 | 1.4 | 3.1 | 0.1 |
| Fruit and Nuts (1 medium apple and 6 almonds) | 92 | 3.7 | 0.4 | 11.7 | 11.5 | 2.2 | 1.9 | 0 |
| Fruit and Nuts (1 medium apple and 2 brazil nuts) | 125 | 7.3 | 1.9 | 11.6 | 11.6 | 2 | 2 | 0 |
| Fruit and Nuts (1 medium apple and 1 tsp nut butter) | 122 | 6.2 | 1.3 | 12.5 | 11.8 | 2.6 | 2.4 | 0 |
| Fruit and Nuts (1 small banana and 6 almonds) | 90 | 3.2 | 0.3 | 12.2 | 10.8 | 1.8 | 2 | 0 |
| Fruit and Nuts (1 small banana and 2 brazil nuts) | 123 | 6.9 | 1.8 | 12.1 | 10.8 | 1.6 | 2.2 | 0 |
| Fruit and Nuts (1 small banana and 1 tsp nut butter) | 121 | 6.2 | 1.3 | 12.8 | 10.9 | 1.4 | 2.7 | 0 |
| Fruit and Nuts (1 medium orange and 6 almonds) | 101 | 3.5 | 0.3 | 13.2 | 13 | 2.9 | 2.5 | 0 |
| Fruit and Nuts (1 medium orange and 2 brazil nuts) | 134 | 7.1 | 1.8 | 13.1 | 13 | 2.7 | 2.7 | 0 |
| Fruit and Nuts (1 medium orange and 1 tsp nut butter) | 132 | 6.4 | 1.4 | 13.8 | 13.1 | 2.5 | 3.3 | 0 |
| Veggies and Hummus (1 carrot and 1 tbsp hummus) | 122 | 8 | 0.8 | 7.3 | 4.9 | 3.8 | 2.7 | 0.4 |
| Veggies and Hummus (1 stick celery and 1 tbsp hummus) | 96 | 7.9 | 0.8 | 2.9 | 0.7 | 1.2 | 2.6 | 0.5 |

| | ENERGY (kcal) | FAT (g) | SATURATED FAT (g) | CARBOHYDRATES (g) | SUGAR (g) | FIBRE (g) | PROTEIN (g) | SALT (g) |
|---|---|---|---|---|---|---|---|---|
| Veggies and Hummus (1 spear broccoli and 1 tbsp hummus) | 106 | 8 | 0.8 | 3.4 | 0.8 | 2.6 | 3.8 | 0.4 |
| Veggies and Hummus (1/2 red pepper and 1 tbsp hummus) | 113 | 7.9 | 0.8 | 5.7 | 3.5 | 3 | 3 | 0.4 |
| Spinach and Mango Smoothie | 97 | 2 | 0.5 | 14.2 | 14 | 2.5 | 4.1 | 0.1 |
| Beetroot and Orange Smoothie | 117 | 0.6 | 0.2 | 22 | 21 | 3.8 | 3.1 | 0.6 |
| Baked Berry Squares | 130 | 3.2 | 0.6 | 19.6 | 6.9 | 2.3 | 4.3 | 0.3 |

# INDEX

A

almond milk, Berry and Chia Smoothie 36

apples 216
    Baked Berry Squares 223
    Spinach and Mango Smoothie 220

asparagus, Teriyaki Salmon and Coriander Rice
    123

avocados
    Cheesy Nachos 196
    Grilled Chicken and Sweetcorn Salad with
        Chilli Cream Dressing 163
    Tomato and Avocado Salad 84

B

bacon, Omelette 39

Baked Berry Squares 223

Baked Ham and Cheese Sandwich 55

Baked Tomatoes with Goat's Cheese 86

bananas 216
    Beetroot and Orange Smoothie 222
    Porridge and Fruit 30

basil
    Caprese Pasta Salad 83
    Chicken and Chorizo Pasta Bake 140
    Curry Beef Noodle Bowl 94
    Fish Pie 194
    Lasagne and Salad 92
    Roast Basil Chicken 157
    Smoked Mozzarella Couscous Salad 176
    Tuna Panzanella Salad 79

BBQ Chicken Salad 78

beans
    Chicken Quesadillas and Salad 149
    Cream of Broccoli Soup 63
    Mini Grill 40
    *see also* black beans; black-eyed beans; green
        beans

beef
    Beef Lo Mein 108
    Beef with Mushroom Sauce and Sweet
        Potato Wedges 200
    Beef and Rice 100
    Buffalo Steak and Corn 109
    Cheeseburger and Fries 201
    Chilli 105
    Cottage Pie 99
    Curry Beef Noodle Bowl 94
    Ginger Beef 97
    Italian Steak 102
    Lasagne and Salad 92
    Meatballs and Spaghetti 103
    Pot Roast 104
    Sizzling Steak Fajitas 188
    Spaghetti Bolognese 96

beetroot
    Beetroot and Orange Smoothie 222
    Goat's Cheese and Beetroot Salad 174
    Mackerel and Quinoa 120

berries
    Baked Berry Squares 223
    Berry and Chia Smoothie 36
    Overnight Oats 33
    Porridge and Fruit 30
    Spinach and Mango Smoothie 220

Best Tomato-based Sauce, The 206

black beans
    Cheesy Nachos 196
    Chilli 105
    Courgette and Corn Chilli 186
    Veggie Burger 202

black-eyed beans
    BBQ Chicken Salad 78
    Cajun-Grilled Chicken and Black-Eyed Bean
        Salad 88
    Fish Cakes and Salad 128

Boiled Egg and English Muffin 32

Breakfast Sandwich 35

broccoli
    Beef with Mushroom Sauce and Sweet
        Potato Wedges 200
    Breakfast Sandwich 35
    Chicken and Loaded-Vegetable Bake 144
    Cream of Broccoli Soup 63
    Five-Spice Chicken 158
    Ginger Beef 97
    Italian Steak 102
    Mango Chicken 145
    Roast Basil Chicken 157
    Stuffed Chicken with Lemon, Capers and
        Chilli 153
    Sun-Dried Tomato Salmon 114

Teriyaki Salmon and Coriander Rice  123
Brussels sprouts, Pork with Sprouts  138
Buffalo Steak and Corn  109
butternut squash
    Butternut Squash and Lentil Curry  182
    Butternut Squash and Vegetable Soup  62
    Fish Cakes and Salad  128

C
Cajun-Grilled Chicken and Black-Eyed Bean
    Salad  88
Caprese Pasta Salad  83
carrots
    Beef Lo Mein  108
    Berry and Chia Smoothie  36
    Carrot and Coriander Soup  66
    Chicken and Ginger Curry  146
    Chicken Kebabs  170
    Chicken and Lentil Soup  70
    Chicken and Loaded-Vegetable Bake  144
    Chicken Noodle Soup  60
    Chilli Salmon Noodle Bowl  126
    Cottage Pie  99
    Herby Roast Chicken  143
    Lasagne and Salad  92
    Mackerel and Quinoa  120
    Minestrone Soup  65
    Moroccan Chickpea Stew  187
    Pork Tenderloin with Orange Marinade  132
    Pot Roast  104
    Roast Basil Chicken  157
    Spanish Chicken Stew with Chickpeas  161
    Spicy Pork and Carrot Stir-Fry  134
    Sweet and Sour Pork  135
    Tantalising Tuna Salad  75
    Veggie Pancakes  172
cauliflower
    Butternut Squash and Vegetable Soup  62
    Chicken and Loaded-Vegetable Bake  144
celery
    Beef Lo Mein  108
    Chicken and Lentil Soup  70
    Chicken and Loaded-Vegetable Bake  144
    Chicken Noodle Soup  60
    Chicken Salad Sandwich  54
    Cottage Pie  99
    Fish Cakes and Salad  128
    Hearty Chickpea Soup  68
    Lasagne and Salad  92
    Minestrone Soup  65
    Smoked Mozzarella Couscous Salad  176
    Sweet Potato and Celery Soup  61
Cheddar cheese
    Baked Ham and Cheese Sandwich  55

BBQ Chicken Salad  78
Breakfast Sandwich  35
Cheeseburger and Fries  201
Cheesy Nachos  196
Chilli  105
Pepper Frittata  177
Veggie Burger  202
*see also* cream cheese; feta cheese; goat's
    cheese; mozzarella cheese; Parmesan
    cheese; ricotta cheese
cherry tomatoes
    BBQ Chicken Salad  78
    Best Tomato-based Sauce, The  206
    Caprese Pasta Salad  83
    Chicken Salad Sandwich  54
    Fish Cakes and Salad  128
    Quick Fish Stew  117
    Spaghetti Bolognese  96
    Tantalising Tuna Salad  75
    Tempting Turkey Salad and Crisp Bread  74
chia seeds
    Berry and Chia Smoothie  36
    Overnight Oats  33
chicken
    BBQ Chicken Salad  78
    Cajun-Grilled Chicken and Black-Eyed Bean
        Salad  88
    Chicken and Chorizo Pasta Bake  140
    Chicken Fajitas  148
    Chicken and Ginger Curry  146
    Chicken Goujons  167
    Chicken Kebabs  170
    Chicken and Lentil Soup  70
    Chicken and Loaded-Vegetable Bake  144
    Chicken Noodle Soup  60
    Chicken Parmesan  162
    Chicken Quesadillas and Salad  149
    Chicken Salad Sandwich  54
    Chicken Tacos  193
    Five-Spice Chicken  158
    Grilled Chicken and Sweetcorn Salad with
        Chilli Cream Dressing  163
    Hawaiian-Inspired Chicken Fingers and
        Sweet Potato Wedges  190
    Herby Roast Chicken  143
    Hot Chicken Sandwich  54
    Mango Chicken  145
    Roast Basil Chicken  157
    Roast Italian-Style Spicy Chicken  159
    Spanish Chicken  152
    Spanish Chicken Stew with Chickpeas  161
    Spinach Salad with Chicken, Corn and Feta  85
    Stuffed Chicken with Lemon, Capers and
        Chilli  153

Tex Mex Chicken and Wholewheat
    Noodles 156
Thai Red Curry and Fried Rice 195
chickpeas
    Falafel 180
    Hearty Chickpea Soup 68
    Minestrone Soup 65
    Moroccan Chickpea Stew 187
    Spanish Chicken Stew with Chickpeas 161
Chilli 105
chilli peppers
    Cheesy Nachos 196
    Chicken Tacos 193
    Chilli Salmon Noodle Bowl 126
    Courgette and Corn Chilli 186
    Curry Beef Noodle Bowl 94
    Curry Coconut Fish Parcel 131
    Grilled Chicken and Sweetcorn Salad with
        Chilli Cream Dressing 163
    Meatballs and Spaghetti 103
    Minestrone Soup 65
    Roast Italian-Style Spicy Chicken 159
    Spaghetti Bolognese 96
    Spicy Pork and Carrot Stir-Fry 134
chorizo
    Chicken and Chorizo Pasta Bake 140
    Granny Brid's Chicken 154
    Spanish Chicken Stew with Chickpeas 161
Cinnamon and Yogurt Pancakes 46
coconut, desiccated
    Curry Coconut Fish Parcel 131
    Hawaiian-Inspired Chicken Fingers and
        Sweet Potato Wedges 190
coconut milk
    Haddock with Coconut Rice 122
    Indian Fish Curry 127
    Thai Red Curry and Fried Rice 195
Continental Fruit Salad 38
coriander
    BBQ Chicken Salad 78
    Cajun-Grilled Chicken and Black-Eyed Bean
        Salad 88
    Carrot and Coriander Soup 66
    Cheesy Nachos 196
    Chicken Quesadillas and Salad 149
    Chicken Tacos 193
    Chilli 105
    Chilli Salmon Noodle Bowl 126
    Courgette and Corn Chilli 186
    Five-Spice Chicken 158
    Indian Fish Curry 127
    Mexican Cod 112
    Moroccan Chickpea Stew 187
    Pork Medallions with Super Green Sauce 137

Seafood Curry 119
Sizzling Steak Fajitas 188
Spicy Pork and Carrot Stir-Fry 134
Teriyaki Salmon and Coriander Rice 123
Tex Mex Chicken and Wholewheat
    Noodles 156
Thai Red Curry and Fried Rice 195
Cottage Pie 99
courgettes
    Butternut Squash and Vegetable Soup 62
    Cheesy Nachos 196
    Chicken and Chorizo Pasta Bake 140
    Courgette and Corn Chilli 186
    Mexican Cod 112
    Punchy Pasta and Roasted Tomatoes 183
    Salmon and Couscous 115
    Turkey Pesto Pasta 164
    Veggie Pancakes 172
couscous
    Chicken Kebabs 170
    Salmon and Couscous 115
    Smoked Mozzarella Couscous Salad 176
    Sun-Dried Tomato Salmon 114
    Tantalising Tuna Salad 75
Crackers and Cheese 214
cream
    Chicken Tacos 193
    Granny Brid's Chicken 154
    Grilled Chicken and Sweetcorn Salad with
        Chilli Cream Dressing 163
Cream of Broccoli Soup 63
cream cheese
    Beef with Mushroom Sauce and Sweet
        Potato Wedges 200
    Crackers and Cheese 214
    Creamy Mushroom Pasta 185
    Mediterranean Breakfast Pitta 45
    Sea Bass with Salsa-Inspired Sauce 110
    Smoked Salmon Roll 214
    Turkey Pesto Pasta 164
Creamy Mushroom Pasta 185
cucumbers
    BBQ Chicken Salad 78
    Chicken Quesadillas and Salad 149
    Goat's Cheese and Beetroot Salad 174
    Salmon and Dill Mayo Sandwich 56
    Smoked Mozzarella Couscous Salad 176
    Tempting Turkey Salad and Crisp Bread 74
    Tuna Panzanella Salad 79
curries
    Butternut Squash and Lentil Curry 182
    Chicken and Ginger Curry 146
    Curry Beef Noodle Bowl 94
    Curry Coconut Fish Parcel 131

Indian Fish curry 127
Seafood Curry 119
Thai Red Curry and Fried Rice 195

E
eggs
Boiled Egg and English Muffin 32
Breakfast Sandwich 35
Chicken Goujons 167
Cinnamon and Yogurt Pancakes 46
Fish Cakes and Salad 128
Fish Goujons 166
French Toast 49
Hot Start 37
Mediterranean Breakfast Pitta 45
Mini Grill 40
Omelette 39
Pepper Frittata 177
Sweet and Sour Pork 135
Thai Red Curry and Fried Rice 195
Veggie Burger 202
Veggie Pancakes 172

F
Fajita Spice Mix 210
Falafel 180
feta cheese, Spinach Salad with Chicken, Corn
and Feta 85
fish
Curry Coconut Fish Parcel 131
Fish Cakes and Salad 128
Fish Goujons 166
Fish Pie 194
Haddock with Coconut Rice 122
Indian Fish Curry 127
Mackerel and Quinoa 120
Mexican Cod 112
Quick Fish Stew 117
Sea Bass with Salsa-Inspired Sauce 110
Seafood Curry 119
*see also* salmon; tuna
Five-Spice Chicken 158
flaxseed/linseed
Baked Berry Squares 223
Continental Fruit Salad 38
Overnight Oats 33
Spinach and Mango Smoothie 220
French Toast 49
fruit
Cinnamon and Yogurt Pancakes 46
Continental Fruit Salad 38
Fruit Cup 215
Fruit and Nuts 216
Porridge and Fruit 30

G
ginger
Chicken and Ginger Curry 146
Ginger Beef 97
Pork with Sprouts 138
Seafood Curry 119
Sweet and Sour Pork 135
Teriyaki Salmon and Coriander Rice 123
goat's cheese
Baked Tomatoes with Goat's Cheese 86
Cheesy Nachos 196
Goat's Cheese and Beetroot Salad 174
Omelette 39
Granny Brid's Chicken 154
green beans
Beef Lo Mein 108
Fish Pie 194
Ginger Beef 97
Italian Steak 102
Grilled Chicken and Sweetcorn Salad with
Chilli Cream Dressing 163

H
Haddock with Coconut Rice 122
ham
Baked Ham and Cheese Sandwich 55
Saturday Night Pizza Special 199
Hawaiian-Inspired Chicken Fingers and Sweet
Potato Wedges 190
Hearty Chickpea Soup 68
Herby Roast Chicken 143
Hot Chicken Sandwich 54
Hot Start 37

I
Indian Fish Curry 127
Italian Steak 102

L
Lasagne and Salad 92
leeks, Cream of Broccoli Soup 63
lemons
Baked Tomatoes with Goat's Cheese 86
Herby Roast Chicken 143
Roast Italian-Style Spicy Chicken 159
Stuffed Chicken with Lemon, Capers and
Chilli 153
lentils
Butternut Squash and Lentil Curry 182
Chicken and Lentil Soup 70
limes
Cajun-Grilled Chicken and Black-Eyed Bean
Salad 88
Chicken Fajitas 148

Chicken Tacos 193
Courgette and Corn Chilli 186
Curry Coconut Fish Parcel 131
Fruit Cup 215
Grilled Chicken and Sweetcorn Salad with
    Chilli Cream Dressing 163

M
Mackerel and Quinoa 120
mangetout, Chilli Salmon Noodle Bowl 126
mangos
    Mango Chicken 145
    Spinach and Mango Smoothie 220
Meatballs and Spaghetti 103
Mediterranean Breakfast Pitta 45
Mexican Cod 112
Minestrone Soup 65
Mini Grill 40
mint
    Fruit Cup 215
    Pea and Mint Soup 71
    Sunshine Salad 80
    Tomato and Avocado Salad 84
Moroccan Chickpea Stew 187
mozzarella cheese
    Caprese Pasta Salad 83
    Chicken Parmesan 162
    Saturday Night Pizza Special 199
    Smoked Mozzarella Couscous Salad 176
    Stuffed Chicken with Lemon, Capers and
        Chilli 153
mushrooms
    Beef with Mushroom Sauce and Sweet
        Potato Wedges 200
    Chicken Kebabs 170
    Creamy Mushroom Pasta 185
    Curry Beef Noodle Bowl 94
    Hot Start 37
    Omelette 39

N
noodles
    Beef Lo Mein 108
    Chilli Salmon Noodle Bowl 126
    Curry Beef Noodle Bowl 94
    Tex Mex Chicken and Wholewheat Noodles
        156
nuts
    Fruit and Nuts 216
    Tropical Muesli Cup 42

O
oats
    Baked Berry Squares 223

Overnight Oats 33
Porridge and Fruit 30
Tropical Muesli Cup 42
olives, Tomato and Avocado Salad 84
Omelette 39
onions
    Beef and Rice 100
    Best Tomato-based Sauce, The 206
    Butternut Squash and Lentil Curry 182
    Carrot and Coriander Soup 66
    Chicken and Ginger Curry 146
    Chicken Noodle Soup 60
    Cottage Pie 99
    Courgette and Corn Chilli 186
    Fish Cakes and Salad 128
    Ginger Beef 97
    Hearty Chickpea Soup 68
    Indian Fish Curry 127
    Lasagne and Salad 92
    Minestrone Soup 65
    Pea and Mint Soup 71
    Pot Roast 104
    Sea Bass with Salsa-Inspired Sauce 110
    Spaghetti Bolognese 96
    Spanish Chicken 152
    Spanish Chicken Stew with Chickpeas 161
    Spicy Pork and Carrot Stir-Fry 134
    Sweet Potato and Celery Soup 61
    Tex Mex Chicken and Wholewheat Noodles
        156
    Veggie Pancakes 172
    *see also* red onions; spring onions
oranges 216
    Beetroot and Orange Smoothie 222
    Berry and Chia Smoothie 36
    Pork Tenderloin with Orange Marinade 132
Overnight Oats 33

P
pancakes
    Cinnamon and Yogurt Pancakes 46
    Veggie Pancakes 172
Parmesan cheese
    Chicken Parmesan 162
    Cream of Broccoli Soup 63
    Lasagne and Salad 92
    Punchy Pasta and Roasted Tomatoes 183
    Stuffed Chicken with Lemon, Capers and
        Chilli 153
parsley
    Baked Tomatoes with Goat's Cheese 86
    Beef and Rice 100
    Breakfast Sandwich 35
    Chicken and Loaded-Vegetable Bake 144

Falafel 180
Fish Pie 194
Hearty Chickpea Soup 68
Italian Steak 102
Spanish Chicken 152
Spanish Chicken Stew with Chickpeas 161
Sunshine Salad 80
parsnips
Chicken and Lentil Soup 70
Herby Roast Chicken 143
pasta
Caprese Pasta Salad 83
Chicken and Chorizo Pasta Bake 140
Chicken Noodle Soup 60
Chicken Parmesan 162
Creamy Mushroom Pasta 185
Lasagne and Salad 92
Meatballs and Spaghetti 103
Punchy Pasta and Roasted Tomatoes 183
Quick Tuna Pasta 118
Spaghetti Bolognese 96
Turkey Pesto Pasta 164
peas
Curry Coconut Fish Parcel 131
Hearty Chickpea Soup 68
Pea and Mint Soup 71
*see also* mangetout; split peas
peppers
Beef and Rice 100
Chicken and Chorizo Pasta Bake 140
Chicken Fajitas 148
Chicken Kebabs 170
Chicken Quesadillas and Salad 149
Chilli 105
Curry Beef Noodle Bowl 94
Fish Pie 194
Ginger Beef 97
Goat's Cheese and Beetroot Salad 174
Granny Brid's Chicken 154
Indian Fish Curry 127
Meatballs and Spaghetti 103
Mexican Cod 112
Minestrone Soup 65
Omelette 39
Pepper Frittata 177
Pork Medallions with Super Green Sauce 137
Pork Steak with Peppers and Creamy Polenta 139
Punchy Pasta and Roasted Tomatoes 183
Quick Fish Stew 117
Quick Tuna Pasta 118
Roast Italian-Style Spicy Chicken 159
Salmon and Couscous 115

Saturday Night Pizza Special 199
Sea Bass with Salsa-Inspired Sauce 110
Sizzling Steak Fajitas 188
Spaghetti Bolognese 96
Spanish Chicken 152
Sweet and Sour Pork 135
Tantalising Tuna Salad 75
Tempting Turkey Salad and Crisp Bread 74
Tex Mex Chicken and Wholewheat Noodles 156
Turkey Pesto Pasta 164
pesto
Caprese Pasta Salad 83
Chicken and Chorizo Pasta Bake 140
Turkey Pesto Pasta 164
pineapples
Sunshine Salad 80
Tropical Muesli Cup 42
pizza, Saturday Night Pizza Special 199
polenta, Pork Steak with Peppers and Creamy Polenta 139
pork
Pork Medallions with Super Green Sauce 137
Pork with Sprouts 138
Pork Steak with Peppers and Creamy Polenta 139
Pork Tenderloin with Orange Marinade 132
Spicy Pork and Carrot Stir-Fry 134
Sweet and Sour Pork 135
Porridge and Fruit 30
Pot Roast 104
potatoes
Buffalo Steak and Corn 109
Carrot and Coriander Soup 66
Cheeseburger and Fries 201
Chicken Goujons 167
Chicken and Loaded-Vegetable Bake 144
Cottage Pie 99
Fish Cakes and Salad 128
Fish Goujons 166
Fish Pie 194
Granny Brid's Chicken 154
Herby Roast Chicken 143
Italian Steak 102
Moroccan Chickpea Stew 187
Pepper Frittata 177
Pork Medallions with Super Green Sauce 137
Pork Tenderloin with Orange Marinade 132
Pot Roast 104
Roast Basil Chicken 157
Roast Italian-Style Spicy Chicken 159

Seafood Curry 119
Stuffed Chicken with Lemon, Capers and
    Chilli 153
protein substitutes 173
Punchy Pasta and Roasted Tomatoes 183

Q
Quick Fish Stew 117
Quick Tuna Pasta 118
quinoa
    Mackerel and Quinoa 120
    Mexican Cod 112

R
raisins
    Chicken Kebabs 170
    Porridge and Fruit 30
    Tantalising Tuna Salad 75
red onions
    Cheesy Nachos 196
    Chicken Fajitas 148
    Chicken Kebabs 170
    Chicken and Loaded-Vegetable Bake 144
    Falafel 180
    Herby Roast Chicken 143
    Moroccan Chickpea Stew 187
    Saturday Night Pizza Special 199
    Smoked Mozzarella Couscous Salad 176
rice
    Beef and Rice 100
    Butternut Squash and Lentil Curry 182
    Cajun-Grilled Chicken and Black-Eyed Bean
        Salad 88
    Chicken and Ginger Curry 146
    Curry Coconut Fish Parcel 131
    Five-Spice Chicken 158
    Ginger Beef 97
    Goat's Cheese and Beetroot Salad 174
    Haddock with Coconut Rice 122
    Indian Fish Curry 127
    Pork with Sprouts 138
    Quick Fish Stew 117
    Sea Bass with Salsa-Inspired Sauce 110
    Seafood Curry 119
    Spanish Chicken 152
    Spicy Pork and Carrot Stir-Fry 134
    Sweet and Sour Pork 135
    Teriyaki Salmon and Coriander Rice 123
    Thai Red Curry and Fried Rice 195
ricotta cheese, Omelette 39
Roast Basil Chicken 157
Roast Italian-Style Spicy Chicken 159

S
salads
    Baked Tomatoes with Goat's Cheese 86
    BBQ Chicken Salad 78
    Cajun-Grilled Chicken and Black-Eyed Bean
        Salad 88
    Caprese Pasta Salad 83
    Chicken Quesadillas and Salad 149
    Goat's Cheese and Beetroot Salad 174
    Smoked Mozzarella Couscous Salad 176
    Spinach Salad with Chicken, Corn and Feta
        85
    Sunshine Salad 80
    Tantalising Tuna Salad 75
    Tempting Turkey Salad and Crisp Bread 74
    Tomato and Avocado Salad 84
    Tuna Panzanella Salad 79
salmon
    Chilli Salmon Noodle Bowl 126
    Salmon and Couscous 115
    Salmon and Dill Mayo Sandwich 56
    Smoked Salmon Roll 214
    Sun-Dried Tomato Salmon 114
    Teriyaki Salmon and Coriander Rice 123
sandwiches 52, 58
    Baked Ham and Cheese Sandwich 55
    Chicken Salad 54
    Hot Chicken 54
    Salmon and Dill Mayo 56
    Turkey Club 55
Saturday Night Pizza Special 199
sauces/dressings
    Best Tomato-based Sauce, The 206
    Super Green Sauce 137
    sweet chilli dipping sauce 190
    Sweet and Sour Sauce 207
    Taco Sauce 193
    Vinaigrette Salad Dressing 209
Sea Bass with Salsa-Inspired Sauce 110
Seafood Curry 119
Sizzling Steak Fajitas 188
Smoked Mozzarella Couscous Salad 176
Smoked Salmon Roll 214
smoothies
    Beetroot and Orange Smoothie 222
    Berry and Chia Smoothie 36
    Spinach and Mango Smoothie 220
soups 58
    Butternut Squash and Vegetable Soup 62
    Chicken and Lentil Soup 70
    Chicken Noodle Soup 60
    Cream of Broccoli Soup 63
    Hearty Chickpea Soup 68
    Minestrone Soup 65

Pea and Mint Soup 71
Sweet Potato and Celery Soup 61
Spaghetti Bolognese 96
Spanish Chicken 152
Spanish Chicken Stew with Chickpeas 161
Spicy Pork and Carrot Stir-Fry 134
spinach
    BBQ Chicken Salad 78
    Berry and Chia Smoothie 36
    Caprese Pasta Salad 83
    Chicken Salad Sandwich 54
    Creamy Mushroom Pasta 185
    Fish Cakes and Salad 128
    Grilled Chicken and Sweetcorn Salad with
        Chilli Cream Dressing 163
    Haddock with Coconut Rice 122
    Hot Chicken Sandwich 54
    Mediterranean Breakfast Pitta 45
    Omelette 39
    Pepper Frittata 177
    Sizzling Steak Fajitas 188
    Spinach and Mango Smoothie 220
    Spinach Salad with Chicken, Corn and Feta
        85
    Tantalising Tuna Salad 75
    Tempting Turkey Salad and Crisp Bread 74
    Tuna Panzanella Salad 79
split peas, Sunshine Salad 80
spring onions
    BBQ Chicken Salad 78
    Breakfast Sandwich 35
    Cajun-Grilled Chicken and Black-Eyed Bean
        Salad 88
    Curry Beef Noodle Bowl 94
    Haddock with Coconut Rice 122
    Pork Medallions with Super Green Sauce 137
    Sweet and Sour Pork 135
    Teriyaki Salmon and Coriander Rice 123
Stuffed Chicken with Lemon, Capers and Chilli
    153
sun-dried tomatoes
    Cajun-Grilled Chicken and Black-Eyed Bean
        Salad 88
    Chicken and Chorizo Pasta Bake 140
    Sun-Dried Tomato Salmon 114
Sunshine Salad 80
sweet potatoes
    Beef with Mushroom Sauce and Sweet Potato
        Wedges 200
    Chilli 105
    Hawaiian-Inspired Chicken Fingers and
        Sweet Potato Wedges 190
    Mango Chicken 145
    Sweet Potato and Celery Soup 61

Sweet and Sour Pork 135
Sweet and Sour Sauce 207
sweetcorn
    BBQ Chicken Salad 78
    Buffalo Steak and Corn 109
    Cajun-Grilled Chicken and Black-Eyed Bean
        Salad 88
    Courgette and Corn Chilli 186
    Fish Cakes and Salad 128
    Grilled Chicken and Sweetcorn Salad with
        Chilli Cream Dressing 163
    Quick Tuna Pasta 118
    Saturday Night Pizza Special 199
    Spinach Salad with Chicken, Corn and Feta
        85

T
Taco Spice Mix 210
Tantalising Tuna Salad 75
Tempting Turkey Salad and Crisp Bread 74
Teriyaki Salmon and Coriander Rice 123
Tex Mex Chicken and Wholewheat Noodles 156
Thai Red Curry and Fried Rice 195
tomatoes
    Baked Ham and Cheese Sandwich 55
    Baked Tomatoes with Goat's Cheese 86
    Cajun-Grilled Chicken and Black-Eyed Bean
        Salad 88
    Cheesy Nachos 196
    Chicken Parmesan 162
    Courgette and Corn Chilli 186
    Goat's Cheese and Beetroot Salad 174
    Hot Chicken Sandwich 54
    Hot Start 37
    Italian Steak 102
    Meatballs and Spaghetti 103
    Mediterranean Breakfast Pitta 45
    Moroccan Chickpea Stew 187
    Omelette 39
    Pepper Frittata 177
    Pork Medallions with Super Green Sauce 137
    Punchy Pasta and Roasted Tomatoes 183
    Saturday Night Pizza Special 199
    Smoked Mozzarella Couscous Salad 176
    Spinach Salad with Chicken, Corn and Feta
        85
    Tomato and Avocado Salad 84
    Tuna Panzanella Salad 79
    Turkey Club Sandwich 55
    Veggie Burger 202
    *see also* cherry tomatoes; sun-dried tomatoes
tomatoes (tinned)
    Beef and Rice 100
    Best Tomato-based Sauce, The 206

Butternut Squash and Lentil Curry 182
Chicken and Chorizo Pasta Bake 140
Chilli 105
Hearty Chickpea Soup 68
Indian Fish Curry 127
Lasagne and Salad 92
Meatballs and Spaghetti 103
Minestrone Soup 65
Pot Roast 104
Quick Fish Stew 117
Spaghetti Bolognese 96
Stuffed Chicken with Lemon, Capers and
    Chilli 153
Tex Mex Chicken and Wholewheat
    Noodles 156
Tropical Muesli Cup 42
tuna
    Quick Tuna Pasta 118
    Tantalising Tuna Salad 75
    Tuna Panzanella Salad 79
turkey
    Tempting Turkey Salad and Crisp Bread 74
    Turkey Club Sandwich 55
    Turkey Pesto Pasta 164
turkey rashers
    Lasagne and Salad 92
    Mini Grill 40
turnips
    Chicken and Ginger Curry 146
    Chicken and Lentil Soup 70
    Herby Roast Chicken 143
    Pork Tenderloin with Orange Marinade 132
    Pot Roast 104
    Sweet Potato and Celery Soup 61

V
Veggie Burger 202
Veggie Pancakes 172
Veggies and Hummus 219
Vinaigrette Salad Dressing 209

W
weekly plans 25–27
weight loss
    alcohol 21
    calories 8–9
    common pitfalls 21–22
    eating out 21–22
    the 80% rule 12, 15, 16, 22, 23
    exercise 11, 12, 14, 15, 23
    food labels 17
    habits 11–12, 14–15
    healthy living habits 12, 14, 15
    holidays 23

the hunger scale 13
motivation 10–11
nutrition basics 16–17
pantry basics 19
planning 18
portions, weighing 21
rules for healthy living 14–15
supermarket tips 19–21
tips 7, 8
triggers 7, 10–11

Y
yogurt
    Berry and Chia Smoothie 36
    Butternut Squash and Lentil Curry 182
    Caprese Pasta Salad 83
    Chicken Fajitas 148
    Chicken Quesadillas and Salad 149
    Chilli 105
    Cinnamon and Yogurt Pancakes 46
    Continental Fruit Salad 38
    Fruit Cup 215
    Lasagne and Salad 92
    Mango Chicken 145
    Overnight Oats 33
    Seafood Curry 119
    Tex Mex Chicken and Wholewheat Noodles
        156
    Tropical Muesli Cup 42